The Crone Initiation:
Women Speak on the Menopause Journey

Girl God Books

Edited by Kay Louise Aldred,
Pat Daly and Trista Hendren

Preface by H. Byron Ballard

Cover Art by Kat Shaw

Girl God Books are also available at discount for retail, wholesale,
and bulk purchase. For details, contact us at support@girlgod.org.

www.thegirlgod.com

Praise for *The Crone Initiation*

"It is time for all of us women to embrace our inner Crone of wisdom and strength as our cycles end. This Anthology is surely the compass to guide us in doing so!"
—Mare Cromwell, Author of *The Great Mother Bible*

"Menopause is a time of great change in a woman's life. It can plunge you into the depths of experience – physically, emotionally, mentally and spiritually. Without a guide, mentor or sisterhood, it can be a rough, isolating and confusing journey. The Crone Initiation brings to light real-life stories from a cross-section of women, ages 40s-80s, who have navigated this passage. Through story, poetry and art, these women provide mentorship, comfort and guidance for this sacred initiation. Through inner wisdom and lived experience, these women bring back the honor and reverence for this return to our most essential self, sovereign and powerful. You will leave this book feeling renewed and with a new perspective and reverence for yourself and this next chapter of your life." —Tabby Biddle, Bestselling Author of *Find Your Voice: A Woman's Call to Action*

"Shrouded in invisibility no more, the Crone's voice is heard loud and clear here: brave, outraged, truthful, fierce. Calling from the depths or from the rooftops, this choir of unique voices sings but one powerful song, that of the Wise One who will be silent no more. A trailblazing song for our present and future Crones." —DeAnna L'am, Author of *Becoming Peers - Mentoring Girls Into womanhood* and *A Diva's Guide to Getting Your Period*

"A feast of women's wisdom that brings into sharp and gentle focus the way we encounter crone energy in our lives and bodies. Informative, emotional, creative and enticing - this book offers a tender and fierce portal into the primordial nature of the Crone." —Carly Mountain, Author of *Descent & Rising: Women's Stories & the Embodiment of the Inanna Myth*

Girl God Books

Mentorship with Goddess: Growing Sacred Womanhood

Mentorship with Goddess is a workbook – a year-long programme – a rite of passage – especially useful for the transition into autonomous adulthood – and also for the menopause journey. The programme can be undertaken solo or as a group. The specific aim is *growing* Sacred Womanhood.

Re-Membering with Goddess: Healing the Patriarchal Perpetuation of Trauma

An anthology of women's experiences of trauma—trauma as a result of patriarchy; trauma perpetuated by patriarchy; and how through personal healing of trauma the Goddess is re-membered, re-embodied and resurrected.

In Defiance of Oppression – The Legacy of Boudica

An anthology that encapsulates the Spirit of the defiant warrior in a modern apathetic age. No longer will the voices of our sisters go unheard, as the ancient Goddesses return to the battlements, calling to ignite the spark within each and every one of us—to defy oppression wherever we find it, and stand together in solidarity.

Warrior Queen: Answering the Call of The Morrigan

A powerful anthology about the Irish Celtic Goddess. Each contributor brings The Morrigan to life with unique stories that invite readers to partake and inspire them to pen their own. Included are essays, poems, stories, chants, rituals, and art from dozens of story-tellers and artists from around the world, illustrating and recounting the many ways this powerful Goddess of war, death, and prophecy has changed their lives.

Willendorf's Legacy: The Sacred Body

Travel through time and discover a world where the fullness of women was both admired and deified. Reclaim your beautiful Goddess body through the rich pages of this powerful collection of art, poetry and essays celebrating our divine inheritance as daughters of Willendorf.

Inanna's Ascent: Reclaiming Female Power

Inanna's Ascent examines how females can rise from the underworld and reclaim their power, sovereignly expressed through poetry, prose and visual art.

Re-visioning Medusa: from Monster to Divine Wisdom

A remarkable collection of essays, poems, and art by scholars who have researched Her, artists who have envisioned Her, and women who have known Her in their personal story. All have spoken with Her and share something of their communion in this anthology.

On the Wings of Isis: Reclaiming the Sovereignty of Auset

For centuries, women have lived, fought and died for their equality, independence and sovereignty. Originally known as Auset, the Egyptian Goddess Isis reveals such a path. Unfurl your wings and join an array of strong women who have embodied the Goddess of Ten Thousand Names to celebrate their authentic selves.

The Girl God

A book for children young and old, celebrating the Divine Female by Trista Hendren. Magically illustrated by Elisabeth Slettnes with quotes from various faith traditions and feminist thinkers.

Complete List of Girl God Books
www.thegirlgod.com

"The Crone has been missing from our culture for so long
that many women, particularly young girls, know nothing
of her tutelage. Young girls in our society are not initiated
by older women into womanhood with its
accompanying dignity and power.

Without the Crone, the task of belonging to oneself,
of being a whole person, is virtually impossible."

–Marion Woodman, *Dancing in the Flames*

"*Who is the Crone?* She is the most dangerous, the most radical,
the most revolutionary woman in existence. Whether in fairy tales
or in consensual reality, the old one goes where she wants to and
she acts as she wishes; she lives as she chooses. And this is all as it
should be. And no one can stop her. Nor ought they try."

–Clarissa Pinkola Estés, PhD, *The Power of the Crone*

Table of Contents

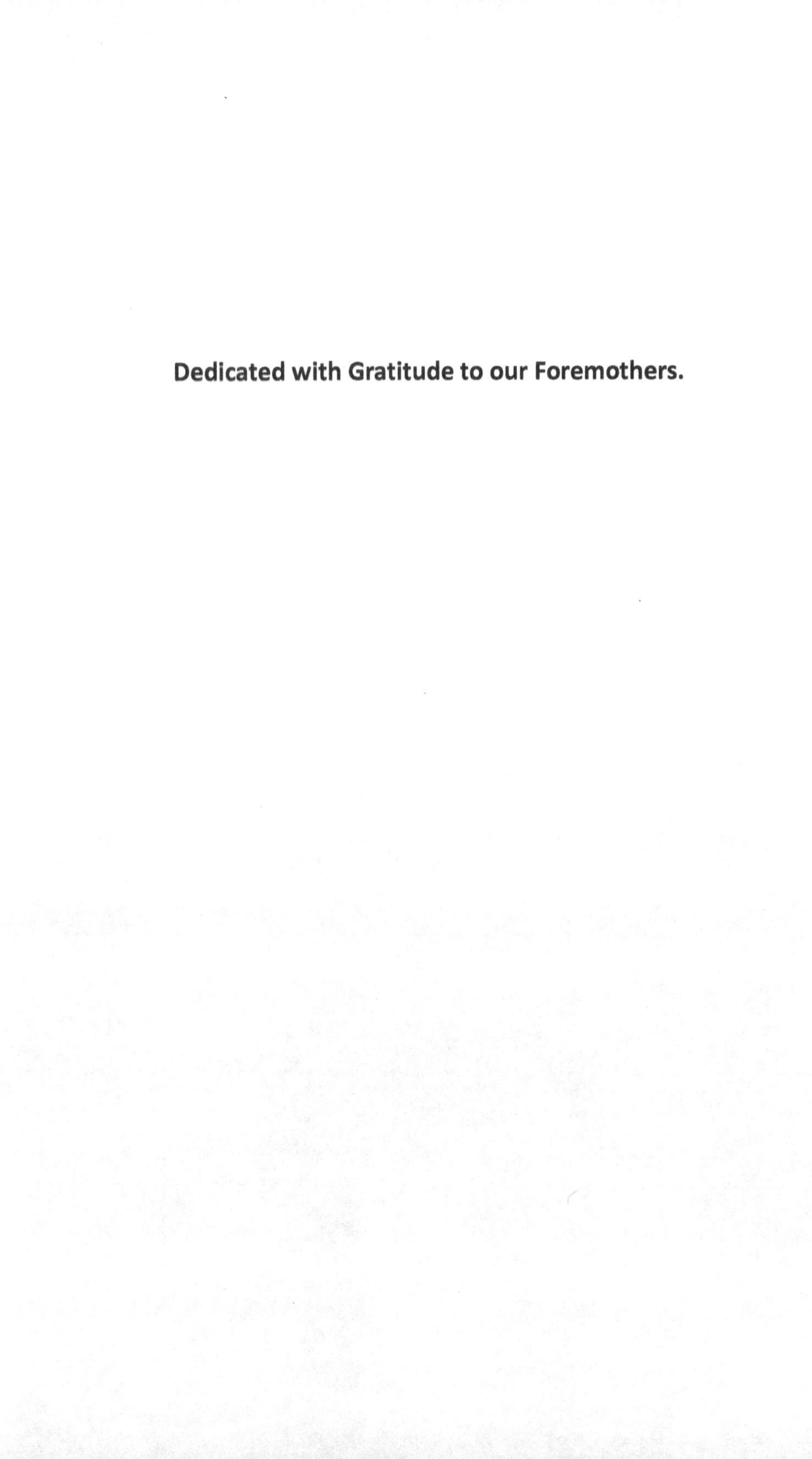

Dedicated with Gratitude to our Foremothers.

Foreword
H. Byron Ballard

O brave new world that has such people in't!
—Shakespeare. *The Tempest*

Hot flashes, forgetfulness, aches and pains and so many more symptoms greet women as we make the extraordinary transition into our Wise Blood Years. "Menopause" is not a big enough word to describe it—we should more rightly think of it as the same process that transforms a caterpillar into a butterfly. Our bodies wrap themselves up and we are stripped of much of what we knew ourselves to be. When the stages are finally complete, we emerge into our magnificent Crone selves—reliant and powerful; answerable to no one except our fine and fierce selves.

Our hormones shift wildly and our Moon times are inconsistent, frightening in their intensity. The culture in which most of us live requires us to soldier on, to continue doing the work we did before, while enduring a physical, mental and spiritual rite of passage. We sweat in air-conditioned offices; we hold our tongues when we want to growl out our impatience with the stupidity that surrounds us. We weep, giggle, mourn, rage. Much of the time, we must also hold this inside. Our behavior must by modulated so that we can retain our clawed-out space in the social structure.

Our mothers could have told us more but they were encouraged to keep silent, too. As we walk these stony paths, we must speak out and tell the story of this walk into a future of power, of wisdom, of keeping the lore. Let us tell our daughters and granddaughters— and also our sisters—what we have learned and are learning on the road to Cronehood.

The writings in this book paint a very different picture than the one we have grown accustomed to—the bent and frail elder who must be treated tenderly, whose memory is faltering, whose best days are far behind her. These are tales of power, of glory, as we rewrite what Cronehood is in this time and embrace the ancient model of authority, wisdom, and resilience. These women teach us to laugh, to sing and to dance. We are reminded of our connection to the broadest cycles of existence and are invited to wield power in ways we have rarely seen modeled.

Crones come to tell us the truth of this time: a truth that has been smothered and hidden for far too long. They pull back the layers of misogyny and ageism to reveal the stunning beauty of the Wise Blood Years, the time of stone and steel, the years of the Witch and the Hag.

Wisdom Keeper
Andrea Redmond

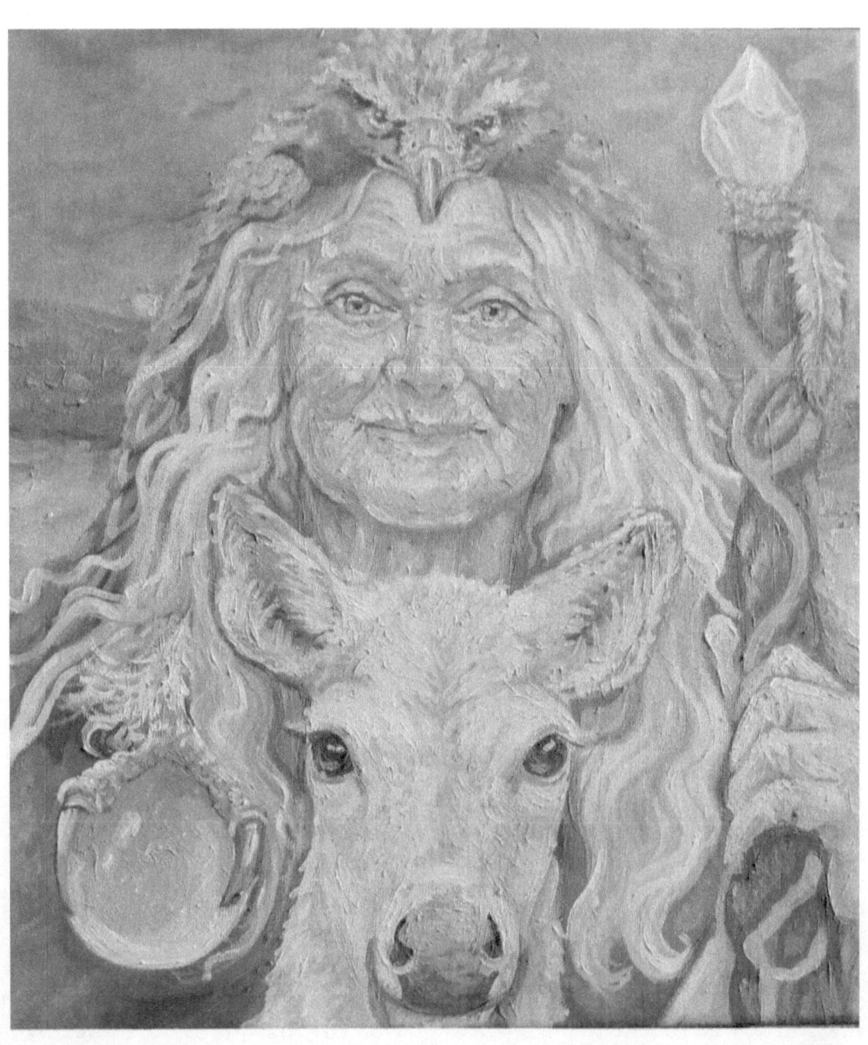

The Crone Invitation and Initiation
Kay Louise Aldred

The Invitation.

When she first arrived in my energy field I was terrified of Crone. I felt her grip on my body and psyche as the breaking down began – hormones and mood spiralling me out of control and togetherness. Her invitation was carried by Jaguar. She waited in the shadows. The envelope was jet black. The writing was jagged and punctuated with ancient symbols, which I later deciphered from runes, and was penned in coagulated old blood and a Crow feather quill I believe. She spoke to me in her obscurity, in a non-reactive and sovereign voice.

"This is an invitation and initiation. You can resist or engage. You can stay and wither or you can journey and thrive. You choose". Fear of the 'lack of control' meant I did resist for several years. As I clung tightly to the old paradigms, ways and layers of Self, body symptoms intensified – hot sweats trying to process the internal rage – and migraines – my splitting psyche unable to hold revelations and knowing and see the conditioning and programming it had been running on. Mood instability was my whole being messaging "YOU. HAVE. TO. CHANGE. EVERYTHING".

And so eventually I said yes to her. She gave me a hand along the way to the yield. Pain. Toxic relationships. A divorce. An exquisite new lover turned soul-full husband. A serious accident. She was insistent. I caved in to be honest. I was on my knees, completely collapsed, already withering at a rapid rate, frail. It turns out saying yes to her invitation is the best decision I have ever made. The breaking down was actually a breaking out – an escape route from falsity, repression and denial. Acceptance was the key which opened the door onto a road of freedom.

The Initiation.

The invitation was handed to me when I turned 37 years old. The initiation itself, also known as perimenopause, seems a lengthy process. I'm still moving through the stages so I can't speak to the outcome, finale or 'end product'. I wonder if there actually is one or if Crone's advancing and closing in is an ongoing undoing of that which is not the truth of Self and of Soul and a taking of the place of 'Elder' and all that means and represents in its fullest and most exalted expression in society.

What I can share is that the most profound and unexpected aspect of the initiation so far has been the igniting of Sacred Rage. Righteous, Holy, Rage. Tapping into this copious lifeforce and allowing it to literally rip through every area of my life, catalysed the onset of the restoration of my boundaries and all aspects of my health. Pure Sacred Rage is savage, indiscriminate, and ferocious. It is the primordial current of Gaia which I've discovered is alive within me. It is not anger. Anger is tempered in comparison and can be channelled, consciously deployed, in many ways.

Sacred Rage is untamed and wild. It has one purpose — to obliterate injustice, untruth, inauthenticity.

As I write this, I can feel this frequency simmering, pulsating, and coursing through my blood. I feel the Earth's annihilating energies and their manifestations — the tsunami, the volcano — and I feel powerful. Crone has gifted me the ability to destroy. I track it moving though me in every hot flush, which are less frequent now that I have plugged into this force. When rage floods my system I pay attention to where I am, the situation and my thoughts, and notice what I need to address, face and change. A devastating demolition is detonated and as I sit in the aftermath — the tatters and ruins — I rest and reflect and wait for the next blitz.

The Crone initiation is not graceful, picturesque or a state of easeful flow. It is not a 'tidy' cyclical experience of letting go gently, making space, planting new seeds, and watching them flourish and grow.

The initiation is brutal, relentless, and thorny. It is barren, barbed, and brazen. Crippling anxiety, the darkest depression, social avoidance, are all part of Crone's training, as she asks time and time again – will you stay the course? She is a no-nonsense mentor, offering tough-love and truth telling. She promises nothing – other than integrity and authenticity. There is no celebration or collaboration and camaraderie in this initiation. It is a solitary path.

About this Anthology
Trista Hendren

The Crone Initiation contains a variety of writing styles from women around the world. Various forms of English are included in this anthology and we chose to keep spellings of the writers' place of origin to honor/honour each individual's unique voice.

It was the express intent of the editors to not police standards of citation, transliteration, and formatting. Contributors have determined which citation style, italicization policy and transliteration system to adopt in their pieces. The resulting diversity is a reflection of the diverse academic fields, genres and personal expressions represented by the authors.[1]

If you find that a particular writing doesn't sit well with you, please feel free to use the Al-Anon suggestion: "Take what you like, leave the rest!" That said, if there aren't at least several pieces that challenge you, we have not done our job here.

Each contributor is on a different part of her journey. The beauty of anthologies is the variety of perspectives they are able to hold within one book. There is no one "right" way to move through menopause. However, we can learn a tremendous amount by listening to what worked—and didn't work—for others.

We welcome you to join us in the circle of 44 women who have shared art or images in this book—as we learn to embrace, nurture, and love the Crone.

---

[1] This paragraph is borrowed and adapted with love from *A Jihad for Justice: Honoring the Work and Life of Amina Wadud.* Edited by Kecia Ali, Juliane Hammer and Laury Silvers.

The Great Initiation
Kay Louise Aldred

Perimenopause, our second adolescence, is a journey which initiates us into our fully expanded and formed 'adult' – our Elder Self – our Crone. It is greater than simply a physical maturation process. Like our teenage years, perimenopause is a complete deconstruction, a dismantling of what is, what we thought of as true, for our bodies, thoughts and emotions, and the birthing of our authenticity, Wise Woman.

We move through the stages of the Great Initiation with Wisdom. The process isn't 'neat'. Detoxing and change rarely are. We purge. We get 'sick', 'hot', 'frustrated'. We have highs and deep lows. We rollercoaster emotionally and hormonally. We face shadows, trauma, pain but also retrieve our gold, medicine and joy.

Personally, as I continue to move through the phases of the admission process, I experience and tolerate extremes I didn't think were possible. I'm burning with rage and passion, despair and ecstasy. Regulation isn't always accessible. The process is untamed and undomesticated. My family is impacted. Cords are cut and attachments severed. My mind, body and energy are pulling back, closing in, reclaiming and taking full ownership of all resources of Self. There is no room in this for other.

It's just me and the Sacred Feminine. Me and my medicine, me and Soul. A process which culminates in Crowning as Triple Goddess.

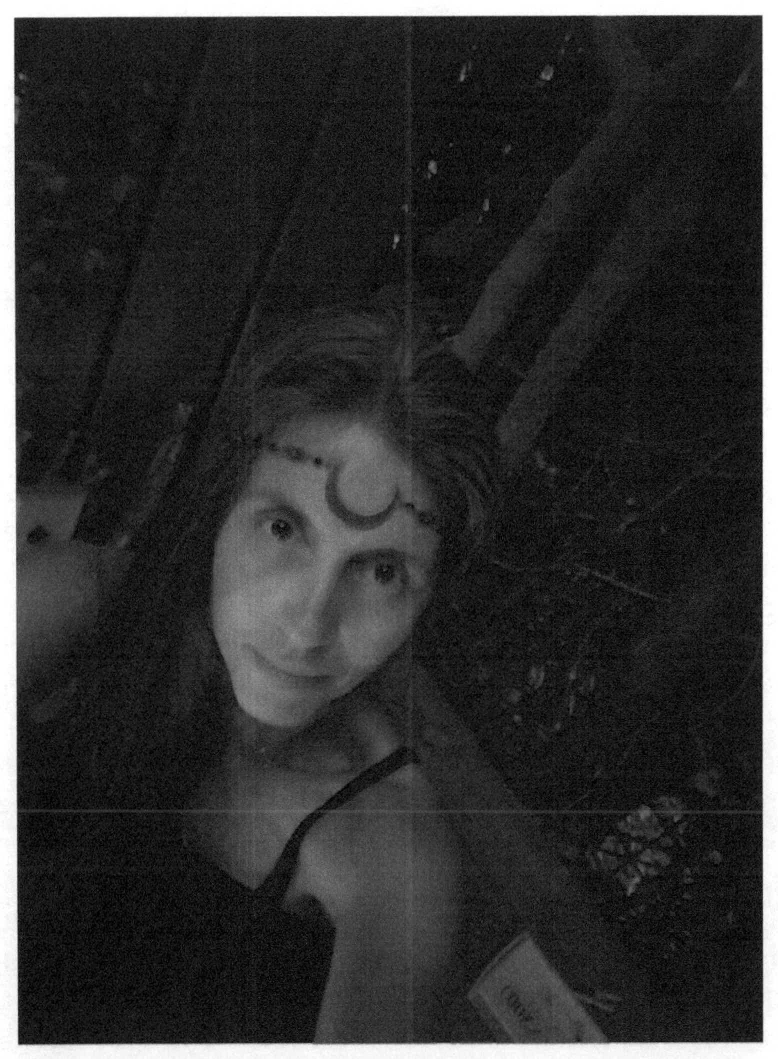

Ceremonies of Consent
and a Declaration of Embarking
Molly Remer

I stood still for a moment,
between bramble and wing,
sunlight on my eyelids
a changing woman
on a changing land
beneath a changing sky...

Perimenopause asks us to make space for dichotomy, not just for our changing bodies, but also with respect to *life.* There is a lot of room for "and" at this life stage, just as with any other stage of a woman's life. Perimenopause is a natural, healthy process full of opportunities for transformation *and* it can be difficult, stressful and confusing. It is important to remember that normal and healthy isn't synonymous only with "amazing and wonderful." Life itself is a normal, healthy process and it can often be painful, confusing, overwhelming and stressful. Pregnancy is a normal, healthy process and it can be challenging, confusing, and with few exceptions, physically changes you forever. Breastfeeding is a normal, healthy process and it can be mysterious, confusing, annoying, and frustrating. Parenting is a normal, healthy process and it can involve the complete deconstruction of personal identity, reforming you into something new in a way that feels painful and soul-destroying while simultaneously being illuminating and soul-evolving. Each of these things can involve distress and the need for help, modification, comfort, and change, as well as still holding the seeds of potential, positive change, and "rebirth" into the next phase of life. Much of life involves both/and, not either/or.

The book *The Seven Sacred Rites of Menopause* explains that perimenopause is a prolonged state of *imbalance*, in which body, mind, and soul work to restabilize, find a new equilibrium, and give birth to a new (or recovered!) self. I find it helpful to see, honor, and hold that imbalance as normal and healthy. Perhaps we can lean gently into the imbalance rather than trying to fix it or ourselves. It is part of this *becoming*, it does not need to be fixed, rushed, or solved. The hormonal shifts of perimenopause create a physical, emotional, and mental between state of transition and change. This time period is not unlike a "second puberty" or "second spring" in which we eventually return to our most essential self, sovereign and powerful, our wisdom in our hands and starlight in our eyes.

This is our undoing.
Unpicking
unraveling
detangling
unsnarling
unraveling loosening
smoothing
freeing ourselves
from the knots we've made around ourselves.
laying down the chains we've gathered
until we are
nakedly alive
alone
unbound.

In the book *The Seven Sacred Rites of Menopause*, author Kristi Meisenbach Boylan draws upon the metaphor of crossing to Avalon as an exploration of what it means to journey into menopause. The journey begins with summoning the barge in perimenopause (at around 40 years old) and concludes with having successfully navigated the misty and choppy waters to the isle of Avalon and the great rite of menopause (at around 52 years old). The process of passing through the Seven Rites is a journey to recover your lost spirit, after which you then take the barge back across the lake and return to the "outer world" again. I think perhaps some women (me included) at this life stage feel concerned that if they draw inward, if they seek solitude and reflection, if they uproot and weed out some of the distractions and unnecessary tasks from their lives, they might be neglecting, overlooking, or letting other people down. In the framework of passing through the Rites of menopause, Boylan asserts that if we are able to give ourselves this time to journey within, we will then be ready to re-emerge into the broader world again—with gifts to offer, wisdom to share, and service to give.

"Finally, I began to write about becoming an older woman and the trepidation it stirred. The small, telling 'betrayals' of my body. The stalled, eerie stillness in my writing, accompanied by an ache for some unlived destiny. I wrote about the raw, unsettled feelings coursing through me, the need to divest and relocate, the urge to radically simplify and distill life into an unknown meaning... Finally, I wrote a series of questions: Is there an odyssey the female soul longs to make at the approach of fifty—one that has been blurred and lost within a culture awesomely alienated from the soul? If so, what sort of journey would that be? Where would it take me?"[2]

"Simone de Beauvoir was of the opinion that if, at menopause, a woman gives her 'consent' to growing older, she is changed into a 'different being,' one who is more herself, one who is complete. I get to my feet and climb down the temple steps, picking my way through the cactus, wondering why we do not have ceremonies of consent."
—Sue Monk Kidd, *Traveling with Pomegranates* (pages 6 and 73)

I came across Sue Monk Kidd's *Traveling with Pomegranates* memoir specifically because another woman referred me to it with the reference of "ceremonies of consent" and I was captivated by the idea that consenting to menopause is a part of the journey and an act of power in a world that conspires to hide the bodies, lives, stories, and wisdom of middle-aged women. I combined this concept with Boylan's metaphor to create a ritual outline for you:

---

[2] Boylan, Kristi *The Seven Rites of Menopause.* Santa Monica Press; 2000.

a ceremony of consent and a declaration of embarking. Different people connect to metaphors in different ways, so you may wish to hold this complete ceremony for yourself, or, you may wish to explore only one aspect of it—a simple statement of declaration, for example—or it may be material you set aside to engage with at a later time. It is up to you!

"But that is what a woman must do when she pulls down the mists around her. She must wrap herself up in her own skin to become the caterpillar in the cocoon. And this securing herself up in her own skin is what facilitates the menopausal process by temporarily closing the veil between her and the outer world."
—Kristi Boylan, *The Seven Rites of Menopause*

Sink my roots into the rich soil
of brave stillness,
drop my heart right down
into the center of everything
where the light of listening is aglow
and the taste of joy is on my tongue...

Summoning the Barge Rite Outline:
Find a private place, ideally near a body of water, but it can even be in your own backyard. Be barefoot, if possible, so your feet can feel the ground beneath you. Also have a glass of water, juice, or tea available.

Before beginning, make a list of women (people) who have inspired you:

Ancestors
Friends
Authors
Artists
Family
Historical figures
Archetypes

Call Your Spirit Back:
Standing by the body of water (or in your own backyard or living room): re-call yourself, re-call your fragments, gather your resources, your reserves, and your strengths to you tenderly, with courage and with love.

If you need more guidance in calling your spirit back, here is an expanded method:

Stand upright with your arms at your sides, palms open. Center yourself in your body, in this time and place, by humming gently as many times as you wish. Visualize your energy field, your spirit or aura. Where is it? What color is it? Where is it extending? Is it reaching into the fields of another person, place, or group? Is it imbalanced or disrupted? Is it vibrant or thinning? Whole or full of holes? Call your spirit in, call your spirit back, from hubbub and bustle and needs and time pressure and to-do's.

Say Aloud:
I call my spirit back
I call my heart
I call my soul
I call my spirit back
I am centered
I am whole.

Put one hand on your heart and one hand on your belly and hum several times again, visualizing your energetic field, your spirit, as whole and completely connected to/surrounding you.

Give Consent:
Then, when you feel settled into your body, into a sensation of wholeness, let the reality of approaching menopause sink into you. And, in this moment, give consent, out loud, for the process to unfold. You may wish to give consent, verbally, three times. You may wish to accompany your consent with sound or movement.

Call upon your ancestors and the women from your list who have inspired you, past or present, living or not. Call upon your inner Wise Woman guide within, your inner Crone and ask them to witness your declaration of embarking.

Symbolically "summon the barge": State out loud that you are summoning the barge, and perhaps even take several steps forward (toward the body of water if there is one).

You may wish to say something like:

This is my declaration of embarking,
as witnessed by my ancestors,
by the wise women who know this path,
by the elements that surround me,
by the courage of my own heart,
by the fortitude of my own spirit,
by the longing of my own soul.
I summon the barge,
I give my consent for this journey,
I set forth.

May I be re-sourced well and wisely,
May I be renewed, rebuilt, and restored,
May I trust my own inner wholeness
To guide the way,
May I embrace the fullness of who I am
May I be open to new discoveries
May I bear witness to change,
Expansion, growth.
May I discover the unexplored terrain of my own being
And may I reach fruitful, enchanted ground.

Seal your rite with a long drink of your water, juice, or tea. You may wish to offer yourself a blessing or affirmation as you drink.

May I be steady,
may I be willing,
may I be bold,
may I walk with patience,
tenderness, grace,
and ferocious determination.

Write, journal, dance, move, pray, sing... however you feel moved to respond to your rite.

It is done.

Additional journal or discussion if working with a group:

1) What would happen if you stopped trying to fix yourself and instead treated yourself/your life stage as simply normal?

2) Does it feel liberating to consider a "second spring" in your life, to think about a "return" to your most core self and to hormonal stability of an earlier phase of your life as you transition into menopause? (Reminder: It is okay if it does not feel liberating—there is no "right way"!)

3) What might you be trying to rush through or force that really just needs time?

4) What leaps are you taking in the dark?

5) Does the idea of "living as a form of not being sure" feel liberating or terrifying to you?

6) If you were to think of your life as a garden, what would you see? What needs tending? What is flourishing and what has withered?

7) What "weeds" are you clearing from your life? What are you releasing?

8) Do you feel a "knot" in yourself? What are you undoing? Do you want to undo any knots in your life?

Message from the Goddess to Those Summoning the Barge
Molly Remer

You are reteaching listening,
you are relearning inspiration,
you are restoring patience,
you are rebuilding joy,
you are replenishing glee,
you are rebirthing delight,
you are renewing what it means
to feel whole
in your own self,
your own body,
your own life.
You are releasing everything
that can be carved away
pared back
surrendered
abandoned
let go.
You are re-calling
yourself,
your spirit,
the ownership
and inhabiting
of your very own life.

Jerusalem Portrait
Liliana Kleiner

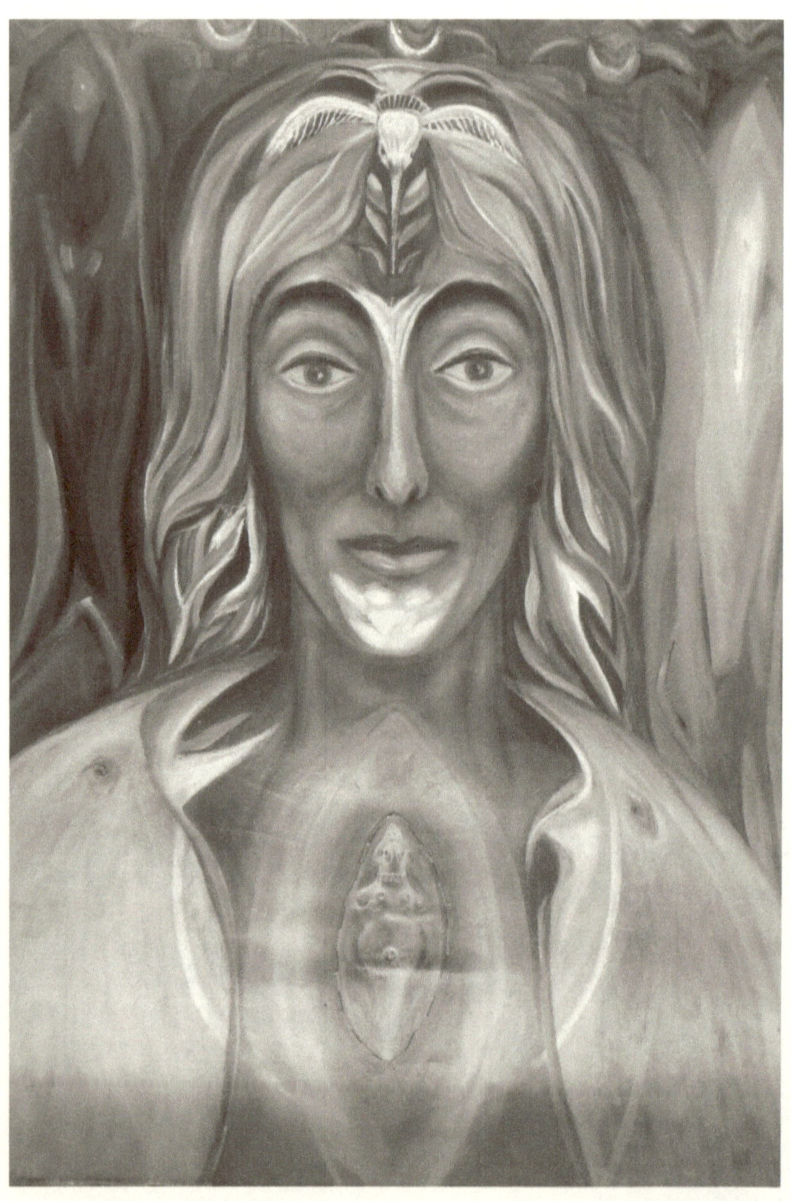

Restorying Menopause:
My Journeys with Inanna, Persephone
and Skeleton Woman
Sarah Miller

Menopause needs a reframe. We need to give this Rite of Passage, this journey of unbecoming and of becoming anew, much more respect and honour. Myth can and does provide a powerful context for restor(y)ing menopause. Goddess myths have a particular potency as they offer powerful motifs of descent and rebirth and hold many keys to our personal and collective navigations through this rite of passage.

The night sweats signalled the beginning of my perimenopausal journey. I would wake drenched with sweat, tangled in cold, wet sheets, after the flush of heat had left my body. Sleep was becoming increasingly difficult, and I had enlisted the help of a Chinese Doctor to assist me. I continued with my life as a passionate and determined activist while navigating perimenopause and then along came ACIS. Andeno Carcinoma in Situ is an aggressive form of cervical dysplasia.

Suddenly I was thrust into the medical system. An immediate hysterectomy was suggested and there was a sense of urgency and fear from the medical practitioners and my family. My response was to slow right down. I hit the pause button on my life and dived deeper into the Mystery of my menopausal journey.

I sought guidance in many different and powerful ways, but the guidance that resonated most deeply was that of myth, those Stories Alive that assisted me on my very personal journey through ACIS, cervical cancer and eventually surgical menopause.

Myths provide a powerful map for journeying through our initiations. Embedded in these tales of transformation we can see repeating patterns, of severance, transition, and return.[3] The stories of Inanna, Persephone, and Skeleton Woman were three powerful Story Guides, offering insights and terrain for navigating my journey through menopause.

Severance

These Goddesses were severed from the life they had known before. Skeleton Woman was thrown over a Cliff, "for she had done something of which her father disapproved." Persephone is either abducted into the underworld, or importantly in earlier myths, She willingly descends. Inanna also goes willingly into the Underworld. Severance through descent is the central to their myths, to their journeys and the transformation that follows. I too would need to descend.

Severance is a separation, a tearing away from. It is psychic, and it is bodied. It is the first part of any initiation, including menopause. In my own journey with ACIS I was stepping deeply into the unknown. I had envisaged a much more graceful journey. But then I had to reckon with this disease in my cervix, and in myself.

At the same time my body was tangoing with the hormonal changes of perimenopause, my 14-year-old daughter was doing her own dance with puberty. She had begun bleeding and was navigating mood swings, and some serious eye rolling, a barrage of whatever's, and an obvious desire to generate distance from me.

It was a painful time and so I turned to the mother daughter myth of Demeter and Persephone. I found recognition in their story of separation, of loss, and of renewal. Their story gave voice to the depth of the grief I was feeling. I missed my young daughter, and the closeness we had. When Persephone willingly journeys to the underworld, "a chill passes through" Demeter. She tries to entice

---

[3] Martin Shaw writes of these phases in his book, *A Branch from the Lightening Tree. Ecstatic Myth and the Grace of Wildness.*

her daughter to stay in the world of sunshine but to no avail. Demeter must face her daughter's departure, this rupture of their relationship, and the beginnings of Persephone's own transformation. She must also face the change that brings for herself.

Their story resonated deeply with me; the grief of letting go and the acceptance and necessity of my daughter's own adventure through her teenage years. I like Demeter was required to step into trust, trusting her to journey well through this difficult period, as she navigated her own hormonal dance of becoming a woman, all the while navigating my own dance.

After being diagnosed with ACIS I journeyed for a year trying to heal myself, and the Stories Alive in my cervical cells. I explored the stories in my body through somatic and shamanic work. I tended to my inner maiden, and the rupture that had occurred in my own teenage years. But 11 months and two cone biopsies later – having declined several offers to remove my womb, I was notified that ACIS had spread from my crypts, and I had cervical cancer. Left unchecked and/or undiagnosed, cervical cancer is a deadly disease. It spreads rapidly through the body. And so I made the painful decision to have a hysterectomy.

With this knowing of my impending surgery I prepared for my departure. In each of these Goddess Myths there are brave souls willing to tend to the Goddesses departure. Inanna has Ninshubar, Persephone has Demeter, and Skeleton Woman has the fisherman. I too called in support. Ninshubar drums for Inanna as she descends into the underworld, and my sisters did just that for me. I also had several womb ceremonies to say goodbye to my womb, to make sacred, this sacrifice of womb to Earth, of menstrual cycling to menopause.

It was also necessary to cultivate my own internal Ninshubar, my witness perspective as I tended to my own ghosts and exiled parts. She sang songs of encouragement as I faced death and bade me honour the life/death/life cycles of which menopause is an important component.

Death is a formidable presence in each of these stories. But it's not only the death of the separate self as proposed in modernity. In these stories death is an integral part of a continuum of death/life/death. Momento mori Skeleton Woman whispered to me. Momento mori, remember you will die. These whisperings were powerful reminders of the eternal cycle within menopause, and in my particular journey.

Like Inanna before me, on that cold surgical table, I was naked and bowed low. My womb, cervix, fallopian tubes, ovaries, and some lymph nodes were cut out of my body. Such radical uncoupling within my bodily self-heralded radical changes in my psyche. This severance is a surrender, a surrendering of who I knew myself to be, and yet these Goddess myths showed me that this was also a process of becoming again.

Transition/Challenges/Initiations

Coming home from hospital I was in an 'in between' place, not here, not there, nowhere really. It was the void, the underworld. This is the place out of which all is born and is restored, but for a while everything is unmanifest. For some time there was nothing to do, nothing really but rest, and trust that my body's illness and recovery are portals to altered states of consciousness, they are ways into this void space. I found it a space of deep embodiment, both of the body and of the void, all at the same time. I found myself more open and permeable to the world alive. The edges of my body were more sharply defined and yet more permeable to sunshine, and rain and wind. Where did my body actually begin and end, what were the boundaries between Her body and mine?

At times I was high on this experience, and on the pain killers. But grief was present too. I had to stay with the grief, tend to all that had already been lost, and for that which I was yet to lose. Like

Skeleton Woman I felt myself tumbling across the deep waters of the seabed, of the feminine psyche. I felt outcast from the "normal passage" through it. I was in what Sharon Blackie calls, "a long brewing in the dark cauldron of transformation."[4] Old griefs, trauma and rage, like characters in an old tale, came to be met. I was meeting the dead aspect of myself, as Persephone does in the underworld. I was meeting my exiled sister/myself as Inanna does and ultimately, I would re flesh myself as Skeleton Woman did.

When all else seemed to be unravelling, I held onto the golden threads of Inanna's, Persephone's, and Skeleton Woman's stories. These ancient and transformational stories were essential to my healing.

While Inanna is lying naked and unconscious on a meat hook (a visceral image for someone who has been through a radical hysterectomy) guides are sent to help her. The kurgarra and galatur attend to the pain of Ereshkigal, the Dark Goddess. And in attending, they heard her cries, and in hearing, they echoed her cries. Ereshkigal is so grateful to be heard that She rewards them with the return of Inanna's body. Listening then provides the necessary integration that will enable her to return transformed from her journey in the underworld.

Similarly in Her story, Persephone willingly goes to the underworld to listen to the "moaning sound" of the bewildered dead. She knows her task is to attend to them, to remind them of their participation in the eternal dance of death/life/death. She "gazes into their eyes" and invites each of them into herself. This merging into Her is a way to return to form, to life, to the manifest.

Menopause offers us the opportunity to listen to the exiled parts of ourselves. To have compassion for all that we are and are not. To be like the Fisherman in Her story and untangle the bones of Skeleton Woman. There was much in me that needed loving

---

4 Sharon Blackie, *The Enchanted Life*, p 108.

attention and listening.

I then had to ask myself what did I want to nourish? What parts of myself needed to be fed? Skeleton Woman knows to fed herself of the fish drying on the racks, Persephone offers the dead the pomegranate seeds and Inanna, well she is given the food of life. Nourishment comes in many forms in these Stories. Yes, it is food, but it is also truth. The truth to be with ourselves, to be with all parts of ourselves and to stay the course, even though we may want to turn and run. It is also the ability to listen, to drink of the tear, and then to embody our truth. And such embodiment requires our return.

The Return

In each of these stories, the return is a powerful process. It is an essential step in reclaiming themselves and integrating and embodying all that they have gleaned in the dark. It is only after drinking from his tear, being nourished by grief that Skeleton Woman reaches deep into the fisherman's body. She pulls out his heart and drums it. His heart becomes a mighty drum, and she bangs out a restorative rhythm. The pulsing of life echoes in her dance and song as she fleshes herself back into being. I too was beating out the rhythms of my heart, singing up the loves for an embodied spirituality, for a World Alive and my place within it.

When we have journeyed well in the depths, in the compost and, in the grief, oblivion and communion, then we too rise rooted.

Like Persephone who returns as Queen, I was finding my own sovereignty.

In their myths the Goddesses are welcomed back. Demeter greets Persephone. Inanna is met by Ninshubar who has kept vigil for three days and three nights, and Skeleton Woman creeps into bed with the fisherman, putting skin against skin. Each showed me the necessity of a very welcome and embodied return.

It takes time to re flesh the body, and longer to re flesh the psyche. My return has been slow but I have the bone-deep recognition that I am not the woman I was before. This journey through menopause, through cervical cancer with these Goddess guides was necessary to help live more fully within cyclical consciousness. To be a voice, a song, a dance of Her reciprocity and "to Body these myths with my own totemic being".[5]

References:

Charlene Spretnak, *Lost Goddesses* of Early Greece, A Collection of Pre Hellenic Myths, Beacon Press 1992.

Wolkstein D and Kramer S, *Inanna Queen of Heaven and Earth*, Harper & Row, 1983.

Clarissa Pinkola Estes, *Skeleton Woman,* (gifted by Mary Uukalat) in *Women Who Run with the Wolves*, Rider, 1992.

Glenys Livingstone, *Pagaian Cosmology, Reinventing Earth Based Goddess Religions*, iUniverse Inc., 2008.

Martin Shaw, *A Branch from the Lightning Tree, Ecstatic Myth and the Grace of Wildness*, White Cloud Press, 2011.

Sharon Blackie, *The Enchanted* Life: *Unlocking the Magic of Everyday*, September publishing, 2018.

---

[5] Charlene Spretnak, *States of Grace*, p143 in Glenys Livingstone's *Pagaian Cosmology*, p109.

Power of Presence
Arna Baartz

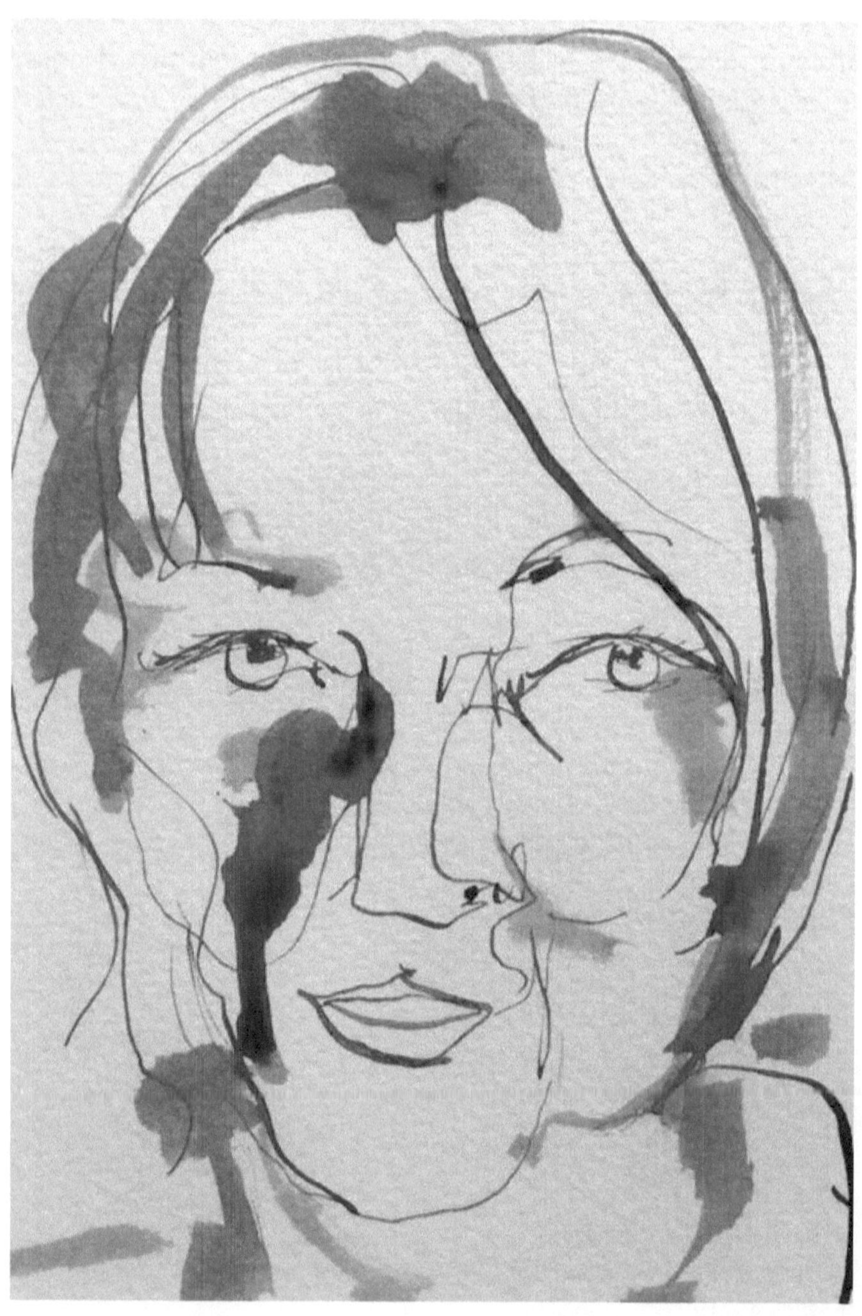

I Turned 50
Arna Baartz

You know my birthday invitation last year read 'help me celebrate 500 years, because 500 sounded easier to deal with than 50.

Really? The things we do for comfort, to blatantly obscure our fear from our self.

I think leading up to the big FIVE OH!!! I was in a kind of active denial... I'm 47 I'm 48 I'm 49 I'm 49.5, 49.6, 49.7...

A furious back-peddling in my mind was occurring as the body hurtled forward into my personal idea of '50', at least into the illusionary construct of life I had created around that number. And yet it WAS only a number, I knew this, I hated myself for even caring about it at all, a hate which only compounded the issue or served to indicate the levels of influence society had had upon me. But I found out as I reached my happy birthday that you can't know what you don't know and as yet I had no true idea of how terrified I was of what came after 50.

I had EVERY reason to be terrified it turned out; I was set to smash head-on into the boundary of all my outdated beliefs. All the bullshit I had packed around me to soften the blows and attempt to control this perceived unsafe world, all the sudden doubt whirled up in a wave of autonomic panic as I outgrew yet another level of the arrogance I'd carefully laid like a slab of sediment during my first 50 years.

It wasn't as though I didn't celebrate the beauty of the more experienced woman, the allure of wisdom that emanates so powerfully from an older, inspiring female. I was not immune! I had fallen in deep love with many an elder feminine. The power of presence and confidence is intoxicating.

My issue was with myself and my soul, whom I'd allowed over millennia to be bound and steeped in a warped social misery, expectations unmet, body changing, an exhausting extinction fear. All things somewhat entangled in the 'aging' process. A quickening of fear as the realisation of 50 gone by hit me.

It was as though I had been living in a bubble of a DO IT do it, achieve achieve, ambitious haze and now something out of my control was emerging to clear the view ahead and that involved seeing clearly the stuff I had pretended wasn't there.

From the day I turned 50 I entered a dark night of the soul, a downward spiral into doubt and uncertainty. I'm an extremely metaphysical kind of person so I could see the hero's journey unfolding before me at the same time as fearing it wholeheartedly. I could see the intentions and spiritual demands I had made for passion and joy being answered in myriad ways by the unconscious as it spewed up my inhibiting fears and old belief systems one-by-one until I was literally drowning in fear and had to do what I had been attempting poorly for the previous fifty...

surrender
Be afraid
Be less than
Be too much
Be ugly
Be unhappy
Be poor
Be wrong
Be old
Be sick
Be alone
Be sad

All the being I had not allowed myself to be as I surfed my emotional body.

And it can only be done one moment at a time. No more lip service to 'authenticity' for me. My nervous system won't allow it. No more sloppy thinking or nasty self-talk—all the old habits are being examined and released in favour of all things love and connection. Spirit and nature have been a buoy on a tumultuous, transformative sea for me, plus old wisdoms, ancient rituals, beautiful words and herbal happiness hormones!!

As I read back over this draft it is hard to believe I'm only 5 months into this metamorphosis and I feel in my heart I've still much much more of myself, fear and joy, to experience.

I stand witness as my body finds its new balance and this miraculous brain puts its mush back together into a conceivable form (hoping for a blue and black butterfly!!).

Peering through the denseness of the old and useless paradigm of fear, I think I see a light bobbing and whispering in the distance, a translucent pink, 'keep your head up, you're going to be just fine...'

She is Changing
Andrea Redmond

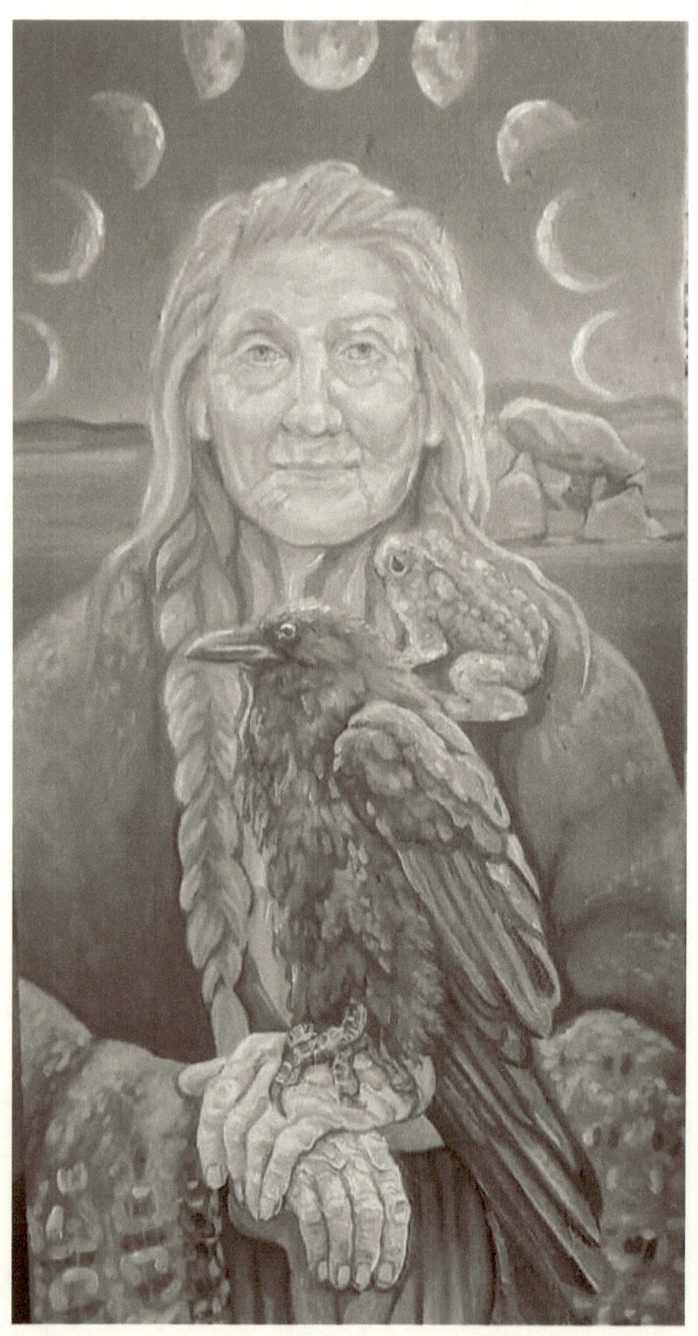

Menopause: Initiation of Sovereignty

Leonor Murciano-Luna, Ph.D.

You are no longer raising your own family, the menstrual cycle has ceased, and you are transitioning into what it means to truly be in your Sacred power and Sovereignty. In the last 5000+ years we have been severed from the Feminine Lunar era as we abruptly entered into the Masculine Solar era, and here the true wisdom of menopause is hidden and even shamed in order to keep women from their power. This is the culture we have been steeped in. And yet all women know deep in their bones, there is a mystery they are biologically and spiritually linked to.

What isn't spoken about is that since the beginning of time, the SHAMANS were really the MEDICINE WOMEN, honored for holding that holy space between the physical and the spiritual, the seen and the unseen. Medicine Women continuously healed individuals and communities through sacred communication with the Earth, with the Divine, acting as that holy channel between the portals of life and death.

Why have women been so denigrated and devalued? Simply because this very inherent power in women that has been persecuted and horrifically condemned for the last 5000+ years, has posed a threat to the power of the domination cultures and their need to control all aspects of life, including the land. But the time has come... all that is changing now... as we awaken to the true Essence of Feminine Consciousness and the holiness that exists within us, within the land and within all of creation.

Menopause is an Initiation, a time of change and a time of Feminine Sovereignty in the life cycle of a woman. It is a time when most women begin to reach the final stages of raising their own families and begin to have more space and time in their own lives. Typically, around the age of forty-nine to fifty-one, is when the journey of peri-menopause begins and when our Initiation begins. Curiously, this time in a person's life correlates with the astrological transit timing of Chiron, the asteroid known as the wounded healer. The themes of this transit in our natal chart represent a time of great transformational initiation that brings up our greatest wound. Chiron essentially signifies our ability to heal and find the true medicine within us, as we move through which 'wounds' are central to our personal life journey. It is a profoundly significant time in our lives and the correlation of the onset of peri-menopause at the same time of Chiron transit in our astrological charts suggests the deep transformation of this time in a woman's life.

In our culture, women are taught to despise and abhor menopause as something distasteful and shameful. The conditioned psychological fear of losing our youthfulness and attractiveness, makes women believe they will lose their value completely. This is because our society values only the 'maiden – reproductive aged women – and denies all gifts related to aging, especially women aging. However, if we take the challenge and realize that our value is not in the superficiality of our looks... the shape of our body... nor in our ability to reproduce... we begin to honor the deeper sacred power that lives in us. If we do not accept the challenge, and we buy into the cultural patriarchal ideology of our worth being tied into our age, we may find ourselves caught in endless depression as those things we identify with our worth change and transform organically. Even worse, we may try to artificially control our biology in the name of 'health' or even 'happiness', both of which are founded on a false idea of who we are and in denial of the natural progression of life, transformation and death. We may be seduced by our misogynistic society desperately trying to sell us all the ways in which we can 'stay young' and be 'valuable', which paradoxically keeps us from the innate power and wisdom of embracing this very initiation of menopause that we may be facing.

As we enter menopause, we enter the space in which we begin our journey into the greater role of Cosmic Mother, no longer just focused on our own children or our smaller circle, but that of greater service to the whole of Earth and her creation. This is the divine role of service that we women are innately here to serve.

And we can look to the MOON as our guide at this time – we have an opportunity to align ourselves, in a greater way, with her cycles and the powerful source of rhythm of the cosmos. With the absence of our own menstrual cycle, we are more intimately connected with the rhythm of the MOON. In the Feminine Lunar era, 5000+ years ago, women were said to menstruate together at the time of the dark MOON. The dark MOON is approximately the three days leading to the new MOON cycle of each month. It is a sacred time of deep inward reflection where we move away from outer focus into the deep focus of the inner realms.

Currently, women have become completely disconnected from their own bodies and their own inner sacredness and usually menstruate during the full MOON (the most yang – outer phase of the moon), due to the fact that we now live in an extremely outwardly (yang) focused culture that denies the inner sacred realities completely. However, in the last 10 years or so, I have seen women menstruating more with the dark moon, especially as they begin to honor their spiritual dimension and the mystery with them. Nonetheless, when we stop menstruating at the onset of menopause, we automatically transition into the greater cosmic cycle and are thus guided by the moon cycle, rather than our own menstrual cycle. Therefore, the dark moon represents our menstrual cycle sacred time to naturally go inward and commune with the sacred mystery within us, receive divinatory messages and align with the cosmic mystery of the Great Mother.

As we enter our initiation, we are being called by the Great Mother and guided by Her representative, the MOON. This is true MOON medicine. The moon moves through the varying frequencies of astrological signs through our sky, as we too are receiving those influx of frequencies and energies on a daily basis – transforming, creating, releasing and regenerating as a service to the Great Mother. We are stars made manifest on the Earth. We are here, embodied beings, playing on this level of physicality and we get to bring heaven on Earth, if we so choose... the more that we are able to honor and acknowledge who we truly are.

This is the wisdom and sacred power of menopause.

The first part of menopause initiation is the peri-menopause, which begins usually between forty-nine to fifty-one years of age, and can continue till about fifty-six to fifty-eight, landing fully in menopause, determined by the absence of the menstrual cycle for at least a year. Every woman is different and these ages can vary, but these are the typical ages we see in general. True Crone wisdom doesn't really set in until we are well-established in menopause and have had a few years completing and anchoring ourselves as wisdom keeper, somewhere between the ages of sixty-five to sixty-nine. But of course, this is a very powerful journey, an initiation into greater service to the Great Mother, anchoring the wisdom here on Earth. This can happen at any age along the way, depending on who we are, and our level of consciousness and service. It is not necessarily a linear process.

Astrologically speaking, we usually have stopped bleeding altogether at the time of our 2nd Saturn return, between ages fifty-eight to sixty, which marks another power stage of our Initiation, woven into this menopause journey. In our 2nd Saturn return, we are truly leaving behind the last thirty years of our life which began between ages twenty-eight to thirty, the previous Saturn return. Between ages thirty to fifty-eight, we have lived mostly in the outer world, involved in child rearing, careers, and outer focus of giving to those loved ones around us. The 2nd Saturn return is a return inward, it is an evaluation and a dismantling of everything we no longer need as we approach the last third of our life. It is a rebirth that is aligned with the deeper true self and with our higher purpose in this lifetime. It is also an opportunity to finally pay attention to our needs fully and give birth to our deepest desires, hopes and meaningful purpose in life. It is a time of stepping into greater responsibility and sovereignty, and of course power that is anchored in our divine dimension.

Physically, the indoctrination of fear and shame of our menopausal stage, in many ways contributes to how we experience the stage of menopause itself, in our bodies and our attitudes.

Many women fear menopause so much that they jump on the bandwagon of taking hormones and other artificial synthetic ways to keep their bodies from displaying their age – maintaining an artificially produced 'younger stage of life' because they fear not having value. Unfortunately, many physicians follow the patriarchal narrative of not honoring the organic process of menopause and fail to see its truer meaning. They are indoctrinated into believing that women's bodies need to be supplemented with artificial hormones in order to maintain health at these ages, which is absolutely not true. Just like in the birthing process, women's bodies are innately designed to move through each stage of life, naturally, and do not necessarily need outside interference in order to survive. Having said that, we may need support at any time in our lives to maintain harmony and create health, but that is very different from believing that the artificial invasive hormonal therapies maintain health in any way. On the contrary, these hormonal interferences stall your body's transitional processes, produce artificially induced periods, dysregulate the delicate organic harmony of hormones, and have been linked with serious health risks, like cancer.

Menopause does not have to have severe symptoms, and the symptoms that you do have are directly related to the state of our bodies and how much we have abused or nourished our self, up to that point. In other words, once we get to peri-menopause, in this time of transition, how we have nurtured or abused our body will be reflected in the quality of transition we have. Greater stress, greater abuse and lack of self-care will present with greater symptoms and dysregulation. Your symptoms also mirror your consciousness, your daily habits, and the overall balance or lack of, that you have kept till that moment. The trauma you have suffered will also reflect on this time of transition. The more abuse on all those levels you have had, and are still having, the more severe your symptoms can be.

Nonetheless, you must understand that your body is in a transition, trying to shift from one stage of your life into another. There are physiological, emotional, mental, and spiritual processes that are taking place in your body. It is a deep initiation and if you have used up a lot of your reserves, then the transition might be a bit rockier.

For example, the hot flashes we see in many women... Think of these as cosmic fires clearing out the mental constructs, narratives and unconscious patterns that are still very active in your psyche, conscious or unconscious, possibly created by trauma in your past. While heat flashes can be purifying, they can also stem from deficiency conditions in your body.

This is also a time of balancing our Feminine and our Masculine energy, psychically and physiologically in our body. So that we can come out into the world... (masculine-yang) rooted in the deep mystery of our soul (feminine-yin). So, our physical body will display wherever our feminine and masculine energies are off balance and needing support, as we transition into menopause.

One of the best herbs to use during this transition is called MUGWORT, artemisia vulgaris. This herb traditionally called 'black sage' can be used on the lower abdomen, sacral chakra area to cultivate and harmonize the yin and yang aspects of your body. It also increases blood circulation and relieves symptoms of menopause, like hot flashes, reported by a study by Pacific College of Health, in 2002. The herb, which can be purchased in a long-rolled cigar-looking stick, can be used to heat various points on the body, being held about 1 inch from the skin (not touching the skin) in the areas of the lower abdomen (CV6, CV4, ST30), ending with the soles of the feet, at the KD 1 point. This method of working and harmonizing women's bodies, called moxibustion, has been used in traditional Chinese medicine for at least 4000 years.

Ultimately, the journey of menopause, beginning with peri-menopause, is a time of great initiation that is marked by several stages of this Initiation, which is always marked by the underlining three stages of all of life: Death-Transition, Transformation and Rebirth.

Death-Transition stage: This is the Chiron initiation at forty-nine, where we start to see the irregularity of the period (peri-menopause). This is where we begin to realize that we are completing a stage in our lives and moving into another stage.

Things begin to change, and we may process the loss or death of one stage (children growing up), as we feel the possibilities and new freedom of a new stage on the horizon. Often, fear accompanies this stage, as we are confronted with the redefinition of 'ourselves' through our roles, values, worth, purpose, aging and even our death.

Transformation stage: This is the stage where we are moving forward on the menopausal journey, experiencing our peri-menopause, releasing, letting go and adapting to the creation of our lives. We may experience symptoms that reflect what is happening in our body and psyche as we transition from one stage to another. Within this stage of transformation, we become a bit more comfortable facing our aging, and the new definitions of our self that we have discovered. We are still in a letting go of the transformational process, but as we release the old, we make space for new strengths, new dreams, new hopes and possibilities to take place. As we prepare ourselves for the new birth, recognizing that it is mostly an initiation of stepping into our power, we will be transforming the places of powerless, unworthiness, inadequacy, doubt and disconnection from the true Essence of our Feminine power. We release and heal from the past wounds of our life and re-establish a new foundation for the rebirth.

Rebirth stage: This is the final stage, and it correlates with our 2nd Saturn Return, which launches us into the last third of our life. As we begin to move into the rebirth, we have a final two years to release the past and move into a new foundation of expression — one that is anchored in our Soul. This rebirth is about birthing our true Essence in greater alignment with our Soul's purpose, in an inner marriage of our spiritual nature and our humanity. This is a rebirth of the inner marriage of Feminine and Masculine qualities within ourselves... where our previous identity is being dismantled and we simultaneously create a new identity that is anchored in the feminine dimension of our being, our soul dimension. As we move out into the world (masculine aspect), we come into greater sovereignty within ourselves, secured in the wholeness of the Universe. This is us living as true human beings, our sacred nature in union with our humanity.

Menopause is a powerful Initiation of Sovereignty for women, where we have an opportunity to grow into our fullness, our wisdom and deep intimacy with source within. This initiation is one of the most powerful initiations a woman has during her lifetime and is truly an accumulation of all the wisdom gathered in her lifetime – and in the collective lifetime of the mothers that have come before her. Whatever transformational work we have done in our lifetime, especially with the clearing of past feminine trauma in the lineage, will start to be evident at this time. And even if we have begun our awakening later in life, we still have the opportunity to transform the wounds that have veiled the women of our lineage, and transform the darkness into light, in this last stage of our lives. Then as we grow into Crone age, we pass on the wisdom we have consciously cultivated to the future generations.

At menopause... women become the Mothers of the Universe... the Mothers of the Earth, a physical representation of embodied spirit in human form, transmitting the true power of being anchored in the source of Great Mother, and acting from the core essence of Love. We have the opportunity to manifest the embodiment of sacredness and holiness in our physical incarnation, in our humanity. This is the gift of menopause, and if we say yes fully to the gift of this stage of our lives, we transform the generational patterns of pain and suffering in the generations that have come before us and that will come after us. We become the living embodiment of the Great Mother herself!

Great Passage from *MOTHER* to *MOTHER WOMB*

Leonor Murciano-Luna, Ph.D.

Who am I now that my children have grown?
Who am I now that I am getting old?
Now... as the tides change and I enter the unknown...
Who am I now?

My life is changing, my body too,
I don't know who I am supposed to be.
The busyness that kept me occupied is no longer part of my day,
No longer do I have to rush off,
From place to place...
Now those that have needed me... have found their own way.

What was once a burden, a challenge, a difficulty,
Is dissolving to the point of non-recognition.
I am freer,
there is new space...
I find myself searching a new experience...
Ahhhh, the bittersweet experience of not being needed.

But the dark Mother calls me... She whispers in my ear...
I know who you are... I see you.

You are now mine,
More fully mine.
It is time to explore the new dimension of being...
A new dimension of seeing.

It is time to liberate yourself from the shackles of the past...
Time to transcend to the depth of the present.
Deep in your womb... is the passage of the mystery.
This is the deep union as the Mother of much more.
You become now the bridge...

the human bridge that is only possible as a soul
that has lived as you have.
Soul in human form that has birthed in human form. You carry the
wisdom that is awakening here, on Earth.
Slowly, you will grow and understand your role
as wisdom keeper, as Crone.
The preparation has begun, and the imprint is in your womb.

You will begin to see with my eyes,
And listen to the whispers of the wind.
You will feel the rhythms of the Moon, and the flame of the Sun.
You will enter the deeper dimension of your womb,
and know the secrets of the mystery...
of the Universe, imprinted there.

Your soul will dance freely in the rain,
as you continue to share your light and your song with the world.
Sometimes quietly,
Sometimes loudly,
But always honestly & truthfully.
You are the voice for primordial Essence of creation.

You are the Universe, dear child...
And now is the time to remember that,
To open to that...
To anchor that in your living experience, on Earth.

This is the time you fulfill the promise of your soul
and lead others to the light of their soul,
This is the role of the Crone,
You become the mother of embodied souls,
Mother to all of creation.
Living in between the worlds,
one foot in each, one breath in each.
As you remember, the world remembers with you.
You are the Mother WOMB.

A Reclamation of Sile na Gig

Andrea Redmond

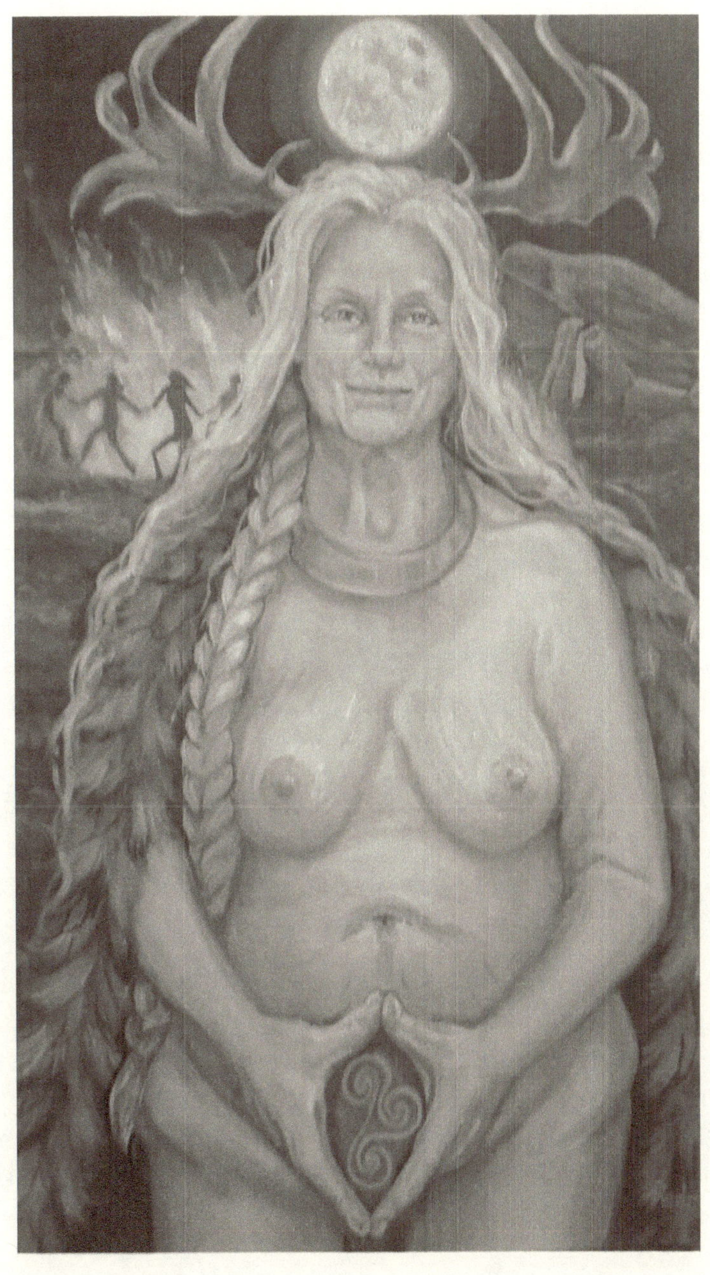

Letting Her In: Welcoming Crone into my Perimenopause

Invocation of the Crone Medicine

Angie Litvinoff

Welcome Crone, embodiment of death and rebirth
Collective nourishment and wisdom
The Void, The Darkness,
The Breaking free of old moulds
The edgy, the unknown, the disconcerting wisdom
The ancestors, the bones, the dance of power
The ashes, the flames, the truth and the voice that says,
'Let go' and 'Surrender' and 'Stop'
Crone, I welcome you, I welcome you, I welcome you!

My perimenopause started with denial.

I was a mother with young children in my early 40's. Surely it wasn't time quite yet? But she had come. And I didn't realise it. I was too much in my head to see it – too busy involved in the lives of others to see what was so obvious on so many levels.

And what she questioned in me was so deep, so profound, so acutely felt, that it was the most pivotal point of my life so far. Truly the great awakening – an aggressive awakening – because SHE was impatient for me. She knew what I needed.

She made me review everything in my life. I mean totally everything. My body was sore, my heart heavy. I had become empty, because what I needed to give to myself, I had given away to everyone else. I had given so much of myself that all that remained was anger. Yes, she activated my liver energy, so that I found the injustice in the way I had chosen to look at life up until that moment.

She began to ask me questions. At first, I took offense. I was annoyed at being challenged. I was too busy pining away for the young woman I was 30 years before. I was mourning and grieving a life I had lost – a life which wasn't real. It was a life I was imagining: the me I was at age 18, 19, 20 but with all the wisdom of an older woman, all rolled into one – a fantasy.

In her wisdom she made me look at myself closely. I began to care for myself, slowly at first, then with a fierce determination. I took a long look at, why had I, for so long, denied myself the right to a place of love in my own life?

My own demons caught up with me. She called them in, one by one, and we began to work through them. She taught me that I don't have to be perfect, that I am whole and complete and enough. Whilst I was beginning a restorative journey of claiming back my energy, I stepped into my Wild Woman and Wise Woman energies at once and left the mother energy behind. I released the habit of over-identifying with her and just took what was right for me. The lesson was this: We don't have to embody all aspects of our archetypes to embrace the aspects we love. We get to choose to identify with what serves us best – that is our right – as women – as Goddesses. We get to choose our identity.

Imagine Crone sitting with me at my side, as I looked at each symptom in turn: as I addressed areas of self-neglect and turned them into strong pride, as I nourished my body with beautiful food, as I began to stretch my body to acknowledge it, and give it love and exercise and as I began to have a routine of self-care.

And as I began to feed my soul with things that brought me joy, I called in a new relationship with creativity, ritual, dance and sensuality.

I began to see my image in the mirror change – not because it had changed – but because my perception of me had grown into a power which Crone was showing me. She was massaging my body, picking out my clothes, healing the hormonal issues and challenges, pointing to me, at me, challenging me to get accountable, to use my skills and my own medicine ways to heal, to ask for help, to say no, to begin to feel my passion again, to cancel things when it all got too much, to stop apologising. To love my wrinkles, stretch marks, my belly and my thighs. To love it all.

It felt effortless and it felt good. I changed my ways and rested. I was no longer a person of service in a role to the world. I became totally and completely Wild Wise Crone.

I no longer mourned for my younger self or felt short-changed. I felt a rising power in me that was proud of the journey and even prouder of the woman I was now.

There was no more chasing, no more running, no more anything.

I simply came home. Crone made a fire, showed me a comfortable place to sit and showed me which way my homeward direction was.

Sitting with love, pain, grief, anger, joy and passion, I birthed the greatest birth I have ever known – the birth of myself.

The letting go led to the rebirth. I let go of all expectations, of approval of others, of seeking praise, of trying to please.

I got focused and began to get grounded: to bring my energies home, to call them back, to beckon my soul parts back. I got my drum – an instrument I feel all women should have – and drummed back my soul parts. I sat alone and drummed – the way I have done for others for so long. I just drummed and felt my own heart open – gently, slowly, gracefully, lovingly.

My heart grew, my resentment lessened, my spirit soared, slowly, gently, softly. I listened because there was silence enough to hear. My parasympathetic nervous system was healing, from burnout, from over giving, from over-identifying with the mother archetype. I had overdone it somewhat but that's OK – I forgave myself and loved myself anyway.

I heard the drum call me deeper into myself, and at first, I sat with the calling just appreciating the rhythm from afar. Then Crone began to move her body and call me closer to the rhythm, to where it was coming from, to the heart of the party. I began to gravitate to where the pulse and the rhythm was and heard so much more: I heard her powerful wail, her celebratory chanting, her rattle. I felt her take my hand and guide me to be right near the pulse, the rhythm, the flow, and I was compelled to move.

Not to any rhythm but my own, Sweet Sister! I felt myself open up to my own pulse, my own rhythm, my own tune, and began to dance a slow dance of recognition – like the dance as your hips open and your cervix gets ready to give birth – that. The dance of the pelvis, the sacrum, the dance of the Creatrix.

I took my time during this rebirthing. Several things were happening at the same time. At first, I was aware of my health and all the changes which pointed to me needing to embrace a level of self-care I knew I deserved, but which I had not embraced right up until now.

This I now understand as a huge part of the inner knowing which occurs in peri-menopause.

At this time, there is a part of you which needs to give yourself a promotion to the Crone Hall of Fame. Our relationship to the world changes. We adapt, so that our outward expression of self is much less about doing the groundwork, it's much more about becoming the architect, the designer, THE CREATRIX. And so, we shift our awareness from merely sowing the seeds and reaping the harvest, to creating powerful intentions very finely with our wisdom and using the grain in new and ingenious ways. Our inside and outside merge. There is no hiding anymore.

We are the wisdom makers and wisdom keepers: the wild ones, the raw ones, the free ones, the liberated.

I began to focus on myself and the ones near and dear to me. More and more joy and understanding began to enter my home. We felt lighter, uplifted, freer than ever before.

I addressed my bleeding gums, my uterine prolapse, my fibroids and heart palpitations, my shedding hair, anger, sweats and weight gain. I gave myself doses of ongoing love, without pressure. I got rid of 75% of my clothes and began to listen to my own needs.

And then I focused on my craft. My medicine became self-expression. I rebirthed as an artist. I embraced my dreams. And the most liberating and powerful aspect of this, is that I found something which was the very first thing in my life that was not reliant on the opinion of others or goal oriented. I create and paint for ITS OWN SAKE. I am not attached to the outcome. I am not attached to the process. I don't care what people think of my art because it makes me so happy. I just LOVE it for it being there for me. I love the fact that it has its own life, its own energy, its own message. It is love on canvass. It is my power.

I felt resistance, reluctance, fear, but I couldn't resist it any longer. The ways of death and rebirth showed me the bare bones of my own life and I created a garden of death, deep inside of me, where I found my newly birthed self.

I looked back at the startling number of encounters with death I have had in my lifetime and took medicine from that too. I took it further and deeper and created an opportunity to review the lessons of life – most recently, just a few months prior to writing this, when I was in hospital on oxygen for days, brushing against death, I got better and painted.

I embraced all that came to challenge me and opened my heart to the true gifts this perimenopause gave me daily. I had never felt so alive – Crone called me to see the beauty in impermanence and to give myself the deepest level of self-respect.

A life review is a total review. So, I also challenged myself to let go of the way I worked, so that I could be nourished by it and adapt to my new way of being – a supportive, kind way. I moved my focus from hands-on to wisdom-led. I invested in myself, with help from others, so I could do this fully supported.

At 48, I could feel my wings unfold as I learned to fly higher than before. Each day is a gift; each breath is sacred.

THIS is her potent medicine.

Lastly and most recently, I acknowledged all my gifts. I let them in and saw myself in my entirety.

And so, I find myself now in a place where I am holding the space for my own transformation. I do this all the time for others, but now is my time. My time to step into the great immersion of soul, to bathe in my own essence, to get to know who I am, who I am becoming and to accept and surrender myself as a 'work in progress perfect being', because I am not striving for anyone else's idea of perfection.

There is no room for the dominant male paradigm – it now clears the way for Crone. I know that my journey is a creative, magical, expressive one. Crone stokes the fire, makes more tea, massages my feet and points in the direction of my dreams, as I sit and hold space for myself with her blessing.

My connection to Crone is also my connection to the elements, to the Earth, to the seasons. She is the season of renewal. She is the element of Earth. She is gritty, deep, wild, wise and beautiful. She is confrontational, creative, powerful, joyful, loving, sassy and truthful. She is free, liberated, light and profound. And she has arrived, Sacred and Divine.

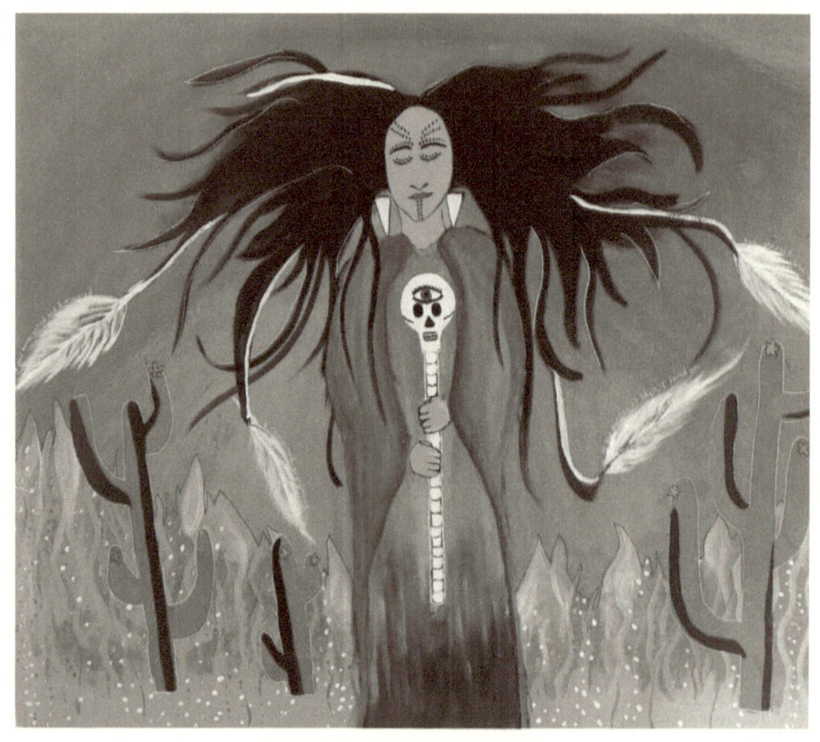

Painting by Angie Litvinoff

No Country for Old Women
Mary Saracino

Howling from the mountaintops
wailing from the riverbanks
scooping the moon into their waning wombs
the old women know that lies kill,
distortions maim, hope isn't enough to feed starving
babies, school the ignorant, put and end to war.

Like Furies, the old ones rise,
clench their furious fists against the blazing sun;
like Harpies they roar, casting dire warnings
upon the winds of change; soothsaying Sibyls
decipher omens, portend the future, speak in baffling koans.
With dakini wisdom they cut through
illusion, vote in primaries, attend caucuses,
raise their voices against power, shatter
the corrupted ceilings that chafe the crowns
of their wizened heads.

The wandering Maenads cry: *"This is no country
for old women."*

Medea calls down her midnight powers,
prays for revolution, strengthens the tired tongues
of memory. Eloquence isn't enough to heal
a wounded country; sequined celebrities
can't mend a nation's odiferous past. Kali avenges
her sisters, the long-patient Queens & Crones,
Maidens & Mothers. The forgotten ones
wait and watch and warn: "Beware the hubris
of ages. Beware the greedy hand that grabs the golden fleece."

Originally published in *She Rises: Why Goddess Feminism, Activism
and Spirituality.*

Things We Don't Talk About at Menopause
Trista Hendren

Trigger Warning for suicide ideation. This was tough to write and may be difficult to read. Make sure you are in a good place first.

After I gave birth the first time, I frantically called the nurse into the bathroom. A brick of blood Jello had plopped out of my vagina— and I was terrified. She just laughed it off and said, *"Oh that's normal!"*

Later, I commiserated with a friend who had a similar experience. *"Why didn't they tell us any of this?"* There was so much about my births that I would do over if I could. Had I birthed another baby, I would have done almost everything differently.

Like birth, menopause is something people don't tell you much about. In my early forties, I began thinking about what books I would read when the time came, but I did not consider that *maybe* I should read them ahead of time to be prepared.

Peri-menopause has been a volatile second adolescence for me. I don't have patience for things I used to. The tantrums I repressed as a child came out in full force. I stopped sleeping well and entered a severe depression.

Nothing about my state of mind made logical sense to me. I had everything in the world to be happy about—but I could not pull myself out of my moods. I tried just about every sort of supplement and herb I could think of before I finally got some relief for my insomnia with Skullcap and Motherwort. But months without decent sleep did a number on my brain—and I could not seem to pull myself out of the hellish anxiety I was suffering. I was embarrassed to tell anyone besides my husband (and finally my best friend) that I sometimes thought about killing myself.

I did not know that suicide idealization in menopause was a thing until I read Susun Weed's book on menopause.

> "Like uncontrollable emotions, thoughts of suicide are normal for menopausal women. Remember that the death phase of menopausal initiation does not imply actual physical death. Yet it would be foolish to deny that the feeling of dying can be as real emotionally as if it were actually happening.
>
> There is a physical/emotional logic to thoughts of suicide. These righting disturbing thoughts can show the menopausal woman the next steps on her journey. Real suicide is an act of desperate self-empowerment. But thoughts of suicide can be pathways to wholeness, health, and self-realization. Like depression, suicidal thoughts during menopause are potent guides to truth and joy."[6]

Wow, I thought! *Why didn't anyone ever tell me this???* I took a screenshot of the passages and sent them to my bestie. She knew instantly this was about me. I thought I had done a pretty good job of hiding it. I didn't want to worry anyone since it seemed highly unlikely that I would go through with it—and I felt self-conscious to be struggling in this way when there was seemingly nothing wrong with my life. It was a huge relief to finally start talking about it. As I opened up to more people, I realized I was not alone.

When I googled *suicidal thoughts during menopause*, I saw a slew of articles that were published last fall.

The Independent reported:

> "Around one in ten women experience suicidal thoughts because of the perimenopause, according to a new study.

---

[6] Weed, Susun. *New Menopausal Years: The Wise Woman Way, Alternative Approaches for Women 30-90.* Ash Tree Publishing; 1st edition, 2002.

Research, exclusively shared with *The Independent*, found around nine in ten women going through the perimenopause experience mental health problems.

The study, carried out by a free women's health app called *Health & Her*, discovered three quarters of women said they had never experienced mental health issues before going through the perimenopause.

Researchers, who polled 2,000 women in the UK aged between 46 and 60 who have experienced the peri-menopause, found just over a third of women polled have not sought help with their symptoms, while eight out of 10 do not discuss mental health issues with their partner or spouse."[7]

Upon reading this, I felt extremely grateful to be married to Anders. This is not my first marriage: I fully understand why so many women do not share this with their husbands.

Weeks later, I came as close as I hope I ever come to taking my life. Anders held me all night while I sobbed until I finally fell into a deep sleep. It was a spiritual death of sorts. I felt the deepest, most excruciating emotional pain I have ever endured in my life. Everything that I had pushed down within me throughout my life was no longer willing to be stored in my body. I couldn't numb it out or stuff it down longer; it wanted to come out.

I realized the next morning that my life was not working for me anymore. In truth, it never had.

I had spent my entire life giving myself away, piece by piece. There was nothing left to give. I had to reassess.

---

[7] Oppenheim, Maya Fear of being labelled hysterical: 1 in 10 women experience suicidal thoughts due to perimenopause Exclusive: 'Many women are suffering in silence, not even talking to their partner or spouse about it,' says expert *The Independent*. 06 October 2021.

And, I had to change.

As someone who abhors any sort of pain, I was puzzled by my sudden desire to slit my wrists. This is the absolute last way I would ever want to end my life. I found Susun Weed's question helpful.

> "If you were to cut your wrists off (cut off your hands, symbolically) what would you no longer have to handle?"[8]

That struck me right at my core. As a recovering co-dependent, I have carried far too many tasks for others my entire fucking life. Carmel Glenane posed a question that has haunted me since I read it several years ago. She wrote, "Delve into yourself and ask yourself why you don't consider yourself 'first' in everything."[9]

The more I thought about it, the angrier I became at my own indoctrination. I find putting myself first almost impossible. And that is after decades of re-programming. While this is frustrating, I think we also must acknowledge that we are deeply socialized since birth to put every single person ahead of our own needs.

When you meet the Crone, She tears down all that nonsense. She demands that Her needs be met first.

I started to let go of things that were not my responsibility. I began to ask for more help. I let go of the energy vampires[10] in my life. I changed my schedule so that it honored me first—and stopped accommodating everyone else to my own detriment.

I began to live on my own terms.

---

[8] Weed, Susun S. *New Menopausal Years: The Wise Woman Way, Alternative Approaches for Women 30-90.* Ash Tree Publishing; 1st edition, 2002.
[9] Glenane, Carmel. "The Alchemies of Isis Embodiment." On the Wings of Isis: Reclaiming the Sovereignty of Auset. Girl God Books; 2020.
[10] Northrup, Christiane. *Dodging Energy Vampires: An Empath's Guide to Evading Relationships That Drain You and Restoring Your Health and Power.* Hay House Inc., 2019.

Susun Weed wrote:

> "If you feel called by death, do not mistake this as a call to take your own life. It is a call to embrace your eventual death as fully as possible while living as fully as possible."[11]

Understanding that these feelings were something that many women experience at this stage of life was deeply affirming to me. I stopped feeling ashamed and selfish—and began to deeply examine what my thoughts meant.

I remember when I read *A Serpentine Path,* I was shocked that the late Carol P. Christ had suffered from suicidal thoughts. After making this connection with menopause, I pulled Carol's book off the shelf once again.

> "I began to understand that the voice that says, *'No one understands me, no one loves me, I might as well die,'* was born in the struggle to suppress my feelings, to grow up, to control myself. Little Carol had never really wanted to die. All she had ever wanted was love. What she needed to say was: *'I hurt, I want, I feel, I am.'*

> Now when I hear the words, *'No one loves me, no one understands me, I might as well die,'* echoing in my mind again—and I will hear them from time to time—I will not be so afraid. I will feel sympathy for little Carol and for big Carol, for whom the struggle to stay in control was just too difficult. I will replace the refrain of ancient pain with the words they masked: *'I hurt. I feel. I want. I am.'* The darkness I feared did not hold a monster. It held a human feeling."[12]

"I hurt. I feel. I want. I am."

Just reading those words brings tears to my eyes. These are radical and affirming words for women.

---

[11] Weed, Susun. *New Menopausal Years: The Wise Woman Way, Alternative Approaches for Women 30-90.* Ash Tree Publishing; 1st edition, 2002.
[12] Christ, Carol P. *A Serpentine Path: Mysteries of the Goddess.* FAR Press; 2016.

I began to acknowledge little Trista more each day. It was easier to love a little girl than a grown woman. It was harder to give my middle-aged self as much compassion in the beginning.

So, I sat with that. And gradually, I began to learn how to love big me too.

It took me a long time to start—and then to finish—this piece. I did not want to share this information about myself. But I have come to realize that I am here today because I *can* share. Suffering alone with these thoughts is torturous.

I want to acknowledge that I am alive today because of the people who have actively supported me. I have a husband and a best friend with whom I can share anything—no matter how dark—without judgment.

Many women do not have such relationships. In the end, in tribute to Carol, I decided to share some of my story too. Her courageous honesty made me feel a lot less alone.

I am also painfully aware that, if I were still living in the United States going through "Family Court" again that my mental state very well could have been used against me. This, I fear, keeps many women silent with their pain.

This must change.

If you find yourself as one of the many women who experience suicidal thinking during peri-menopause, this advice from Ellen Bass was useful to me during my darkest night.

> "If you've tried everything you can think of and you still feel like you can't make it through the night, sit down in a chair and don't get back up. It might be the most miserable night of your life, but morning will come and you'll be alive without having hurt yourself."[13]

---

[13] Bass, Ellen and Davis, Laura. *The Courage to Heal: A Guide for Women Survivors of Child Sexual Abuse*. William Morrow Paperbacks; 4th -20th Anniversary edition, 2008.

These thoughts occur for some of us. They are scary as hell. And, like most things, they will pass.

As I was finishing this essay, I had a long lunch with one of my dearest friends in Bergen who is about a decade younger. She mentioned that she wants to read this anthology because she wants to be prepared when the time comes for her. I told her I was writing this piece, and she said something like, *Yeah, but that isn't going to happen to someone like you.* I saw the tears gather in her eyes as I told her that it already had.

I don't think many of us fully *feel* how precious we are to our friends and family. In that moment, I did.

May we all embrace our inherent Divine worth.

The Crone. Her Light Shines for All
Katrina Stadler

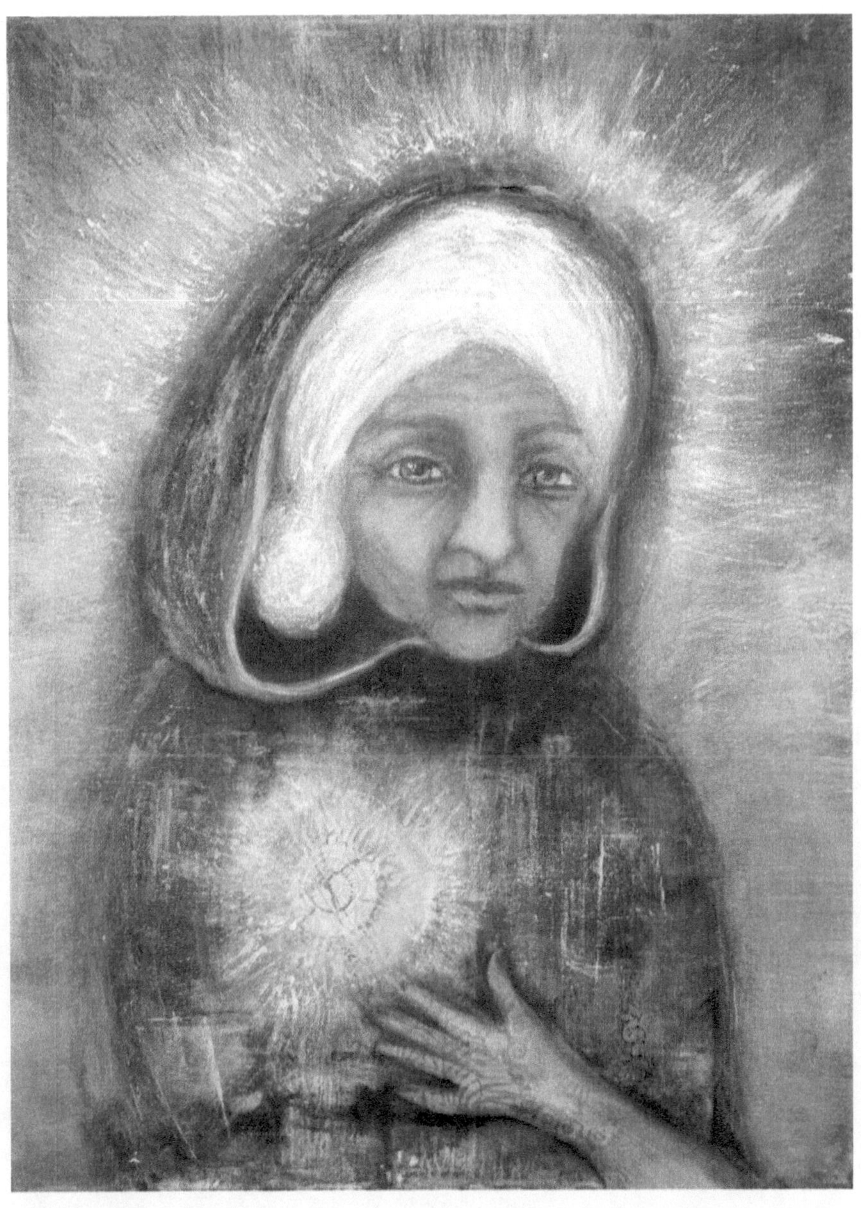

Menopause Magick!

Rebekah Myers

Yes, there are hot flashes
down to your toes,
But this is your power surge
everyone knows.

Yes, there are aches and pains
sleeplessness too,
But these are all birthing
a powerful You.

Yes, there are times
when you feel you'll explode,
But these are to teach you
to lighten your load.

Yes, there are mood swings,
and brain fog and sweats,
But these usher in
your most queenly days yet.

Once all your power
flowed out and away,
But now it flows inward
to strengthen and stay.

Once you felt pressured
to please and to serve,
Now you'll feel freedom
and pleasure, and verve.

Once you felt fearful
of all the unknown.
But now you rejoice!
You are Matriarch, Crone!

© Rebekah Myers, 2022

Matriarch

Rebekah Myers

Matriarch
Maker
She who creates
She who forms worlds

Matriarch
Leader
She who knows
She who paves the way

Matriarch
Harvester
She who reaps
She who gathers

Matriarch
Sovereign
She who is empowered
She who knows herself

Matriarch
Queen
She who reigns
She who has triumphed

Matriarch
Survivor
She who has passed through the fire
She who rises from the flames

Take Your Seat
Mary Lane

It's easy to dismiss a woman who has traveled through the
darkness over and over throughout a long life.

Mastering death and rebirth in order to survive,
within a society that deems it terrifying.

What to do with women who have "remembered" who we are,
quietly in the shadows?

As the maiden and mother step back to honor her in the autumn of
her life.

We take our seat at a table with honor, embracing the wisdom
garnered only through the Divine journey laid before us.

We plant the seeds and nourish the growth of the next generation,
just as nature would do.

We wear our scars, wrinkles, saggy skin, gray and white hair with
grace, dignity, and a knowing that we carry something within our
beings that only we carry, and this world needs.

Wise women, you have earned your seat at the table.

Please take it.

Self-Portrait - Androgyne
Liliana Kleiner

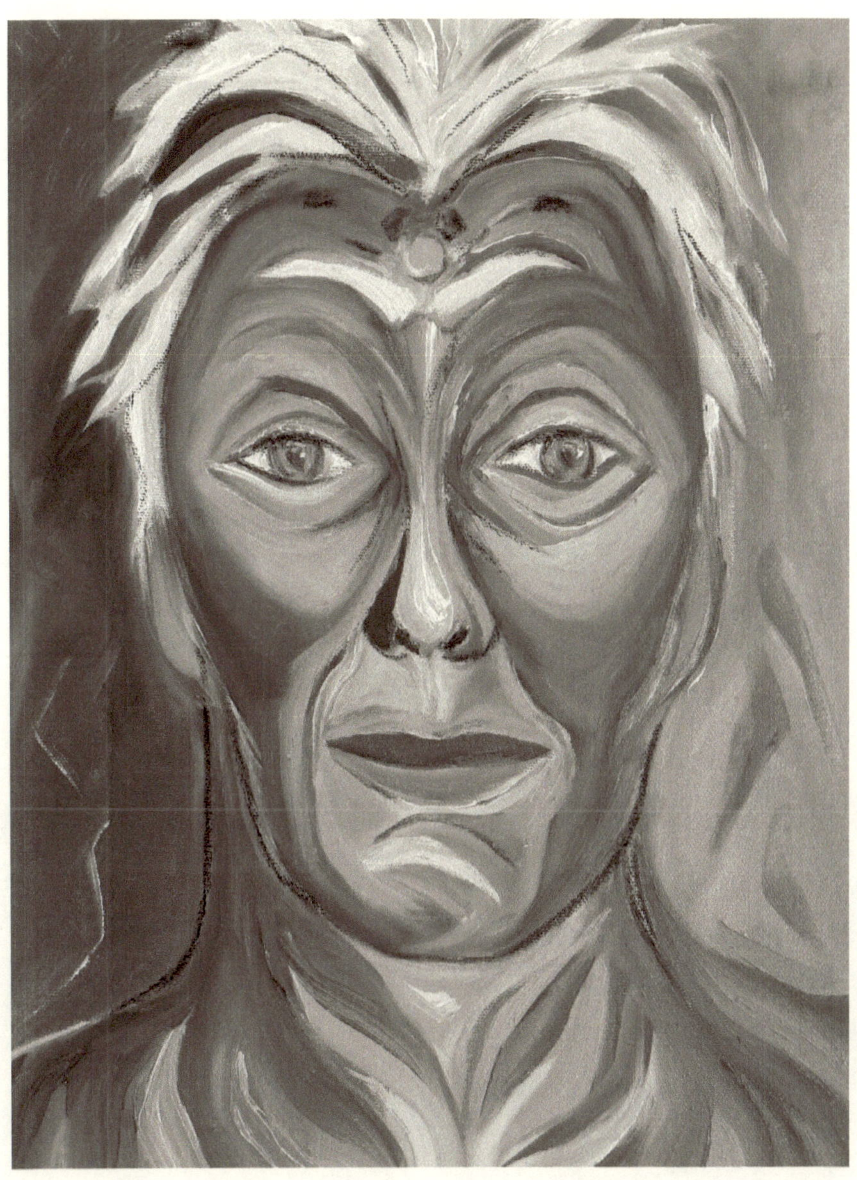

My Crone Years
Stephanie Mines

And the fire in my soul burns as if I were just born.

Is it only the beauty of my words that are left for me?

I wear them like bracelets for my healing hands.

My shadow on the forest floor meets me.

She bends down while my spirit ascends.

I defy the manipulation of this decaying culture, but

Of what value are the protests of an old woman who writes poems

Begging people to rise up?

O my dying country,

You sacrifice your brilliance for cheap toys.

Still, I cry, "My God it is you who has delivered me for these times."
So, I will not shut up or shut down.

I am yet the star child brought forth

For some hidden redemption

In that ropey, tangled under sand of the forest floor

Made by the wanderings of my people,

Down there in the dusty tunnels

With the infinitesimal creatures we depend on, there Is my
salvation, my family that

Cultivates my stubborn entelechy.

Our Lines
Arna Baartz

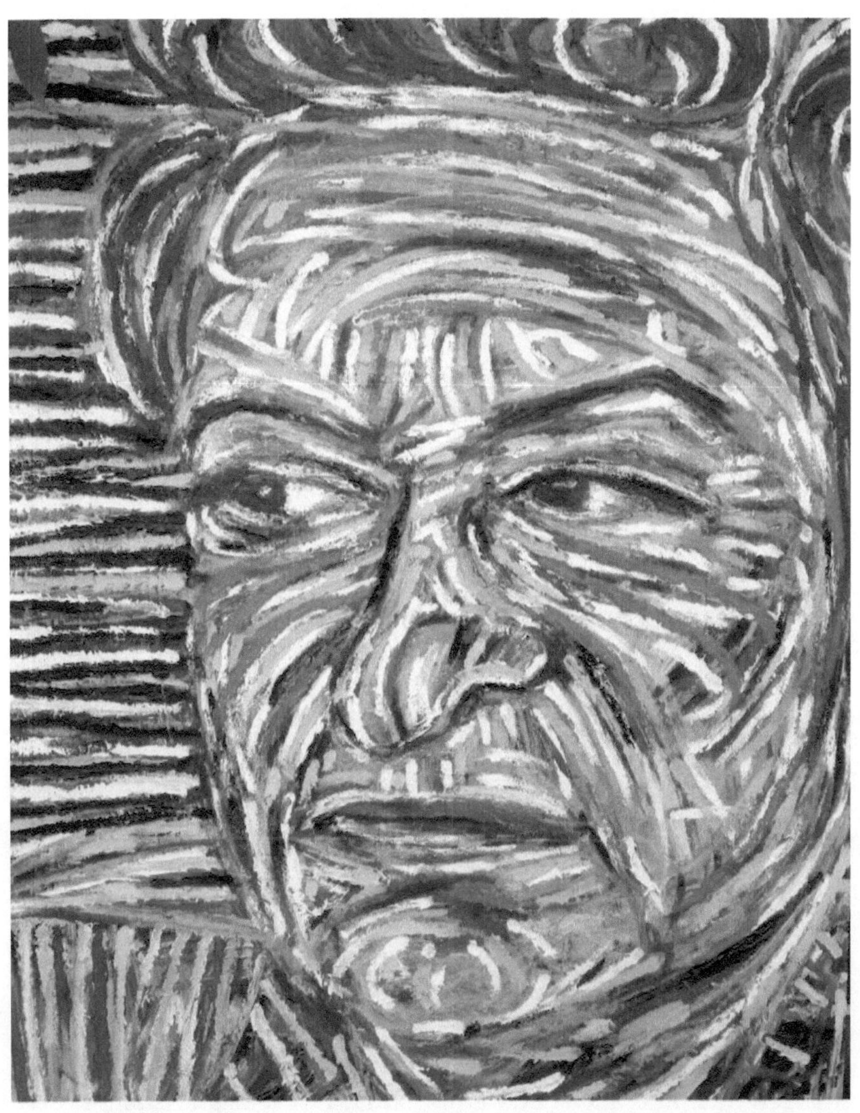

The Culturally Supported Menopause
Catherine Hale

Last night I woke up 10 times.

Despite wanting more sleep I started my day at 5:30 AM. Based on recent months this was a good night's sleep.

You may ask what's going on?

No I don't have a newborn baby to look after. No I'm not ill. No I'm not surrounded by noisy neighbours.

Most nights, for the last 2.5 years, I've been woken by night sweats – surges of heat rising through my body – only to be replaced moments later by icy chills.

In the daytime they come out of nowhere – disabling me mid-task – temporarily paralysing aspects of my cognitive function.

And no – contrary to popular reaction it's not funny – I'm not laughing.

It's exhausting.

Its relentless.

And sometimes it's enough to make me curl up in a ball and cry.

Welcome to menopause.

The third and final act in the trifecta of hormonal initiations women meet after menstruation and motherhood.

Wrapped in layers of social taboo, associations of witches with pointed hats and spells and ample doses of fear and shame – we do our best to avoid talking about it.

I understand.

To acknowledge menopause requires us to meet the fragility of our human existence. By stepping through its doorway we're one step closer to death – and god forbid we talk about anything to do with death.

In a Peter Pan culture obsessed with preserving youth we're told its far better to just pretend everything is all right and we are just doing fine – thank you very much.

Yet right now there are millions of women facing the ordeal of a culturally unsupported menopause on a daily basis.

These are women who are mothers, sisters, wives, lovers, employees, employers and entrepreneurs.

These are women who are, more likely than their male counterparts, working in the caring professions as teachers, doctors, therapists, practitioners and body- workers.

These are women who've been told to get back to work and be 'productive' members of society after they bore children.

These are women who in their bleeding years were told period pain is normal and should just be accepted even if it reduces you to a vomiting wreck each month.

These are women who've lost their voices as their cyclic bodies are forced to live in a linear world.

These are women who may be far removed from knowing what they need, have challenges with receiving because they've been taught to put everyone else's needs first, so they behave in ways that may look like they are just fine as they solider on through each day.

Don't believe it.

It's an act women have been taught to perform.

It's adaptive behaviour stemming from nervous system dsyregulation. It's behaviour which ensures safety and belonging to a culture where female bodies are sexually commodified, where the pay gap between male and female bodied people invites financial dependence, where women's health receives considerably less financial support than male health and where women can still be raped and told it's their own fault for wearing a skirt that was too short – or for not running away.

Seriously...

So when women reach menopause they're probably exhausted, stressed, overworked from living in this exploitive culture and now they don't have their hormones supporting them to carry on with business as usual. Once that oestrogen starts dropping the veil of accommodation slips away and the truth of living in a culture of extraction meets women head on.

At this point dear sisters –

No longer can we wear the superwoman cape.

No longer can we say yes when every part of our body is screaming no.

No longer can we overwork – even when our culture dictates that's the norm.

No longer can we put up with anything that smells like b*llshit.

No longer can we tolerate living in a culture of inequality, injustice and blind ignorance to the environmental disaster that is happening.

And it's scary as hell to realise this. If we change, our belonging is threatened – for will we still be loved if we say no? Will it be safe to speak up when our voices have been historically silenced? Will we still be loved in our ageing bodies when we've been sold the lie of needing eternal youth?

It takes a warrior of a woman to journey through the initiatory fires of menopause. It takes an even stronger community to hold her and to collectively unpack the culture of oppression and supremacy that maintains inequality and to co-create the new world where we are in right relation with all of life. I choose to celebrate each and every woman on this journey for her courage and stamina as she navigates this path in whatever way she has chosen for herself.

So if you know a woman who's in the menopausal age range – including perimenopause – which could be anything from age 35ish - 65ish (although it can happen earlier than this) what are the small and doable steps you can take to offer support and let her know you care?

Maybe you could:

- Let her know that she will still be loved for having and expressing her needs even when historically she's never expressed them before.

- Let her know you respect her need for space by honouring her boundaries.

- Let her know you respect her need for more understanding and compassion when her hormones are fluctuating so much she doesn't know who she is anymore.

- Let her know you respect her need for letting the old version of herself die and the new one be reborn in its place.

- Let her know you'll support her need to change all her routines even if it means you'll see less of her.

- Let her know you'll support her need for more body work/therapy and emotional support.

- Let her know you'll support her need to probably radically change her diet.

- Let her know you'll support her need to let go of what doesn't work for her — even if it ends your relationship.

- Let her know you'll support her need to express the truth she sees so clearly that others aren't able to see.

A conscious and supported menopause grows wise, heart-centered women who've worked through their trauma. They become our natural leaders, guided by truth and a commitment to protect the sacred.

Where you offered her love, you watered the seeds of her worthiness to grow. Where you gave her space to rest, she created natural rhythms of care that honour her body. Where you offered her choice — she knew she was accepted. Where you honoured her boundaries, she knew she mattered.

Let us become the society that holds, honours, and respects these sacred transitions in women so may we all benefit from the labours of their initiation and may this reverence create the beautiful world we all know in our hearts is possible.

Self-Portrait – Arbutus
Liliana Kleiner

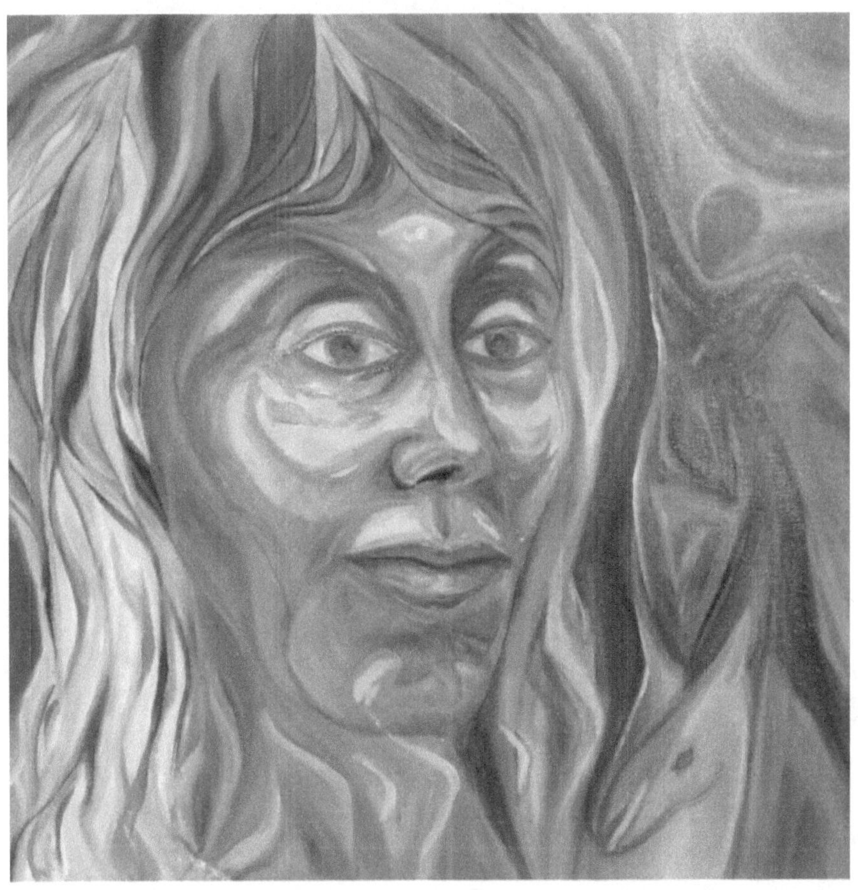

Labels, Paradox and Schrödinger's Cat: Menopause as Sovereignty

Arlene Bailey

Though not an absolute, for many of us there will come a point in time when we question our reason for existing. What is the purpose of our existence... day-to-day and in the larger scheme of things? If we choose the moment to begin breathing, are we not as entitled to choose the moment we stop?

I have reached this moment or rather the cessation of my moon blood has made me feel I've reached this point. There is silver in my hair and my hands and face reflect the tracks of time. I'm not an old woman, though no longer young either and definitely beyond society's demarcation labeled middle age. I have by society's standards outlived my usefulness in that I can no longer bear children (as if I ever could or even wanted to) and am beyond the employable demographic, though also not yet old enough to be considered eligible for Medicare or full retirement benefits.

I am no longer a label. It's as though I am invisible with no maps and NO idea who I am or what comes next. Maybe, though, it's perhaps more as though I exist in a superposition[14] outside the realm of that quantifiable idea of time... outside the realm of observer influence where my behavior equals a demographic which equals a label. Like Schrödinger's Cat,[15] I'm neither dead nor alive or more like I could be either depending on who looks.

Except no one is looking.

---

[14] The principle of superposition claims that while we do not know what the state of any object is, it is actually in all possible states simultaneously, as long as we don't look to check. It is the measurement itself that causes the object to be limited to a single possibility.

[15] Named after Physicist, Erwin Schrödinger.

A small voice says... Wait. You seem upset about that. Hasn't that always been the goal for those who never wanted to fit the mold, never wanted to be defined?

Hmmm... got a point there. When I was a label, easily identified and put in the round hole, I wanted no part of it. I still want no part of it and, yet, there is a certain comfort/sanity/order in standing up and saying hell no I am not part of your little orderly labeling system as opposed to standing there unnoticed thinking hey, did you forget about me over here? – I'm still living, breathing, able to contribute and make a difference so why do you no longer care for what I have to offer?

Hmmm... contradiction... uhhhh, no, paradox. I was something and hated it, but now that I'm not that something, not anything... not a thing, I hate that. WHAT?! Is that what THIS is all about? Feeling as though I no longer exist and it's time to stop breathing because I'm no longer something society notices and hence no longer quantifies? That's FUCKING crazy!

Uhhh, yeah, I've been called that... recently and a lot! It IS crazy. I never wanted to be assigned to a group with a descriptive moniker that implied what my actions and thoughts or abilities were at any given moment in time, based on my skin color, age, where I lived or any of a number of seemingly inconsequential attributes, especially those that said I was a woman because I bled and/or could bear a child. FUCK NO! But I also don't want to be ignored as though this orderly grouping of atoms no longer vibrates in a meaningful way.

Wait, so you want to be measured so as to prove your existence? Don't you realize that by being ignored, not being measured, no societal expectations as to what you should be or not be doing, you exist in all possible states simultaneously!

Hmmm...

Menopause brings the strangest musings and the most unexpected gifts and has taken me down the proverbial rabbit hole more than once. When I was a bleeding woman I could become a mother, both acceptable labels to the status quo. Once I entered menopause, I became an enigma, something society could not label and therefore out of bounds as far as ascribing purpose or usefulness. What do you do with a woman who no longer fits the traditional mold of what patriarchal culture defines a woman to be? How do you wrap her in expectations when you can't see value? You don't. You simply ignore her. Pretend she doesn't exist. Turn your back and walk away unaware of her power building in front of eyes that cannot see.

I have begun to feel I am the phoenix lying only as ash, waiting for that moment when the newly formed head pushes forth breathing its first breath of new, fresh air. Then suddenly, realizing I have wings, I burst forth and take off. No longer with any labels or expectations, I am new energy, transformed into anything I want to be. Holding my wise blood in, I am no longer a measurable or controllable entity.

After all, if I am Schrödinger's Cat – with my life or death (or mere existence) dependent on who is observing – AND if no one is looking and I own that I'm the only one who sees me, the only observer whose opinion matters – then my life, my labels can be whatever I observe/desire them to be. No longer dependent on outside observers to define me, I am free.

Holy Hell. I can be whomever and whatever and they'll never see me coming.

Now that is sovereignty.

Hmmm... Menopause as sovereignty. Now that is a concept and label I can embrace.

Caveat... I wrote this piece 10 years ago as I was exiting my very unique journey of menopause.[16] Although I was about to turn 60 and enter my seventh decade, I in no way felt I was a Crone nor that the holding of my wise blood within automatically made me a Crone. Though many attempted to place that moniker upon me, it simply did not feel right.

I am now 69 with the knowing that 70 (and the beginning of my eighth decade) is not far behind. There has been much wisdom come in these past years and, it is only now that I feel ready to accept the crown of the Crone as I feel her wisdom pulse through every inch of my beingness.

---

[16] See my other article "Unnatural Medical Menopause at 29: How I Reclaimed this Right of Passage" on page 140.

Wisdom's Three
Arlene Bailey

Priestess, Sorceress, Wise Woman, Death

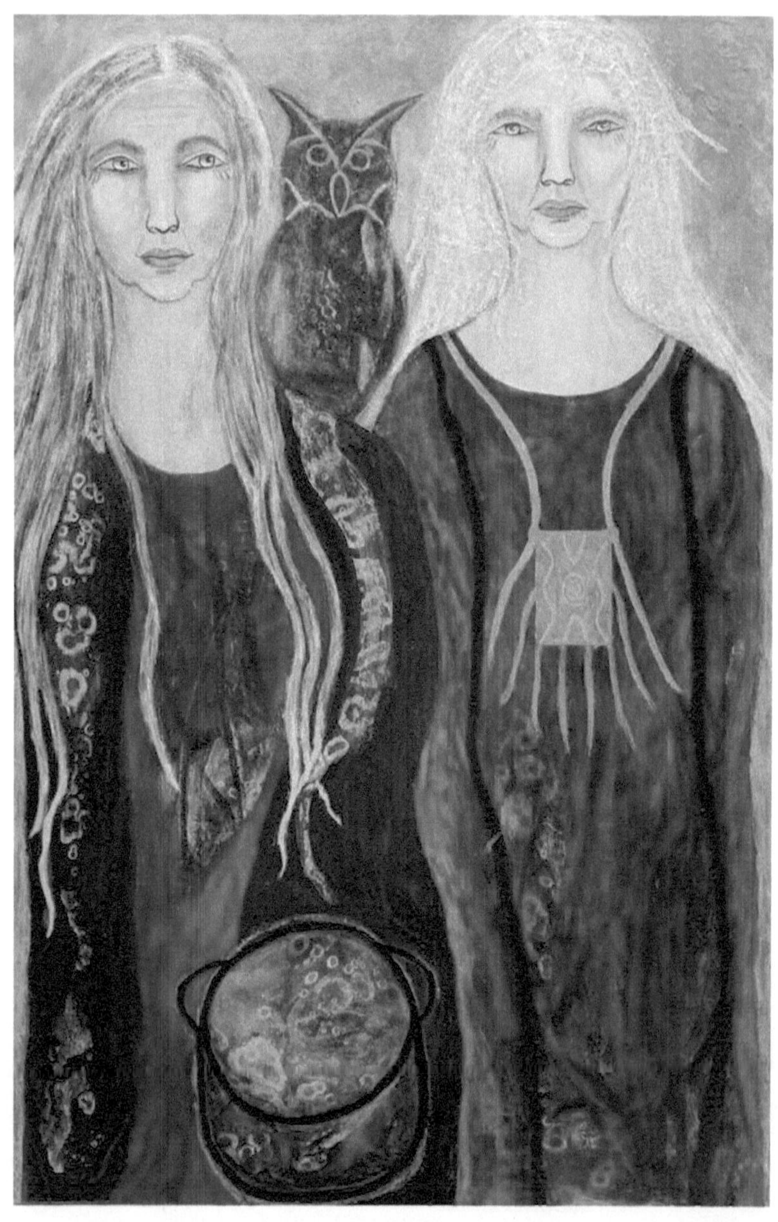

Mother Becoming Crone
Arlene Bailey

As I surrendered to the portal that is the canvas... stood there painting, deeply immersed in where to go next, how to move and going through change after change after more change... the Old Crone always pushing me, guiding me and eventually speaking through me... her words became both manna and warning.

She Speaks...

The Medicine Woman and Priestess stand here remembering their first blood and the ending of their bleeding. They stand here remembering the years between their menopause and when they began to feel my stirrings, my prompts, my guidance and even my admonitions that they would know when it was time to step fully into their version of Crone.

While your Crone lives within from the time you enter this realm, She does not automatically show up just because you no longer bleed and there is no set timeline for each woman is different. In those 'tween years you will walk the Edges, feeling Her just out of your grasp, seeing glimpses but knowing your time of this new embodiment... the time of full presence... is still yet to come for there is much to learn. So as you see into other worlds, gaining new gifts and abilities, turning deeper within and travelling those pathways and ley lines previously unknown and unseen, you listen and you watch and you learn.

AND...

When She does arrive, Look Out!! She will shift you and change you, turn you inside out until the day you realize you are now Crone and the fulfillment of the ALL of woman. You are Priestess and Wise Woman, Sorceress and Hag... you are the young woman with her first blood and you are the Old One walking the worlds of the living and the beloved dead. In fact, more and more you will be the Wise Woman and Priestess of Cosmic Wisdom, walking in Other Worlds, seeing beyond this world's temporal existence until finally you embody the wisdom of the Death Mother and Death Mysteries.

Until this time, things are not static, and you are not simply standing still as you grow and change within while preparing a space for Her. Find your allies (human, animal and cosmic), rely on and trust them for they bring wisdom not heretofore available. Then one day you will realize something has shifted. You have shifted and you now viscerally feel your Crone stirring as your wise blood is held deeper within. You realize the releasing of it back to the Mother is a distant memory, for YOU have transitioned to Crone and your role has shifted from that of birthing – be that children or career – to the wisdom of the ages and the mysteries of the Veil. Now as you walk closer and deeper with the mysteries of this last stage of life, your visions become different and stronger, your words more poignant as is the wisdom you impart. You have entered a realm where you have an understanding of the All of the All – known only in this time to those women... those Crones... who walk on toward the Death Mysteries learning the language of the Veil.

Until that time, however, remember...

Remember, Embody and Embrace the cessation of your moon blood... embrace the time of transition, new learning, and new wisdom... And, when She does show up, embrace that you are Crone and there is much you have to share.

The Moon from the Porch
Annie Finch

The moon has dusks for walls,
October's days for a floor,
crickets for rooms, windy halls.
Only one night is her door.

When I was thirteen she found me,
spiralled into my blood like a hive.
I stood on a porch where she wound me
for the first time, tight and alive,

till my body flooded to find her:
to know I would not be alone
as I moved through the tides that don't bind her
into womanhood, like a flung stone.

With each curve that waxed into fullness
I grew with her, ready and wild.
I filled myself up like her priestess.
I emptied myself like her child.

Flooding, ready, and certain,
I hid her—full, fallow, or frail—
beneath each long summer's rich curtain.
It covered her face—the thin grail

that delivers me now. Now I'm with her.
All the cast shadows come home.
I stand in these shadows to kiss her
and spin in her cool, calming storm.

Now as I move through my own beauty
and my shadow grows deeper than blood,
oh triple, oh Goddess, sustain me
with your light's simple opening hood.

The Priestess
Annie Finch

Hiding a hand is easy in my folded
robes; my whole body is hidden. But the moon
glows where my foot has touched her. And two pillars
open into stone petals near my crown.
And the folds in my robe fall down like water,
and the flames in my candles swell out like grain,
and the hovering words leave me like rain.
Could this quiet birth hold the Earth's old daughter?
I keep the wisdom to carry my own crown.

Sand and Bone
Annie Finch

We came shivering, knowing how lines of the tide
will use seaweed, and sea-drift, and sea-wrack (and bone)
to etch with. We wait to be marked on the sand
(a thick sagging rockweed, its bulbed grace undone),
moved each way like feathers, dragged slow as a hand,
or just whitened — past breath. We'll be moved till we're gone
to where no earth is ready to hold us inside—
(as we follow gull-shadows back over the land).
(We are hiding ourselves where there's no room to hide.
Now we whiten our hair in the wind of no dawn!
Now the seagulls are whitening too!
Now they're born In our turning and turning!

Cailleach
Andrea Redmond

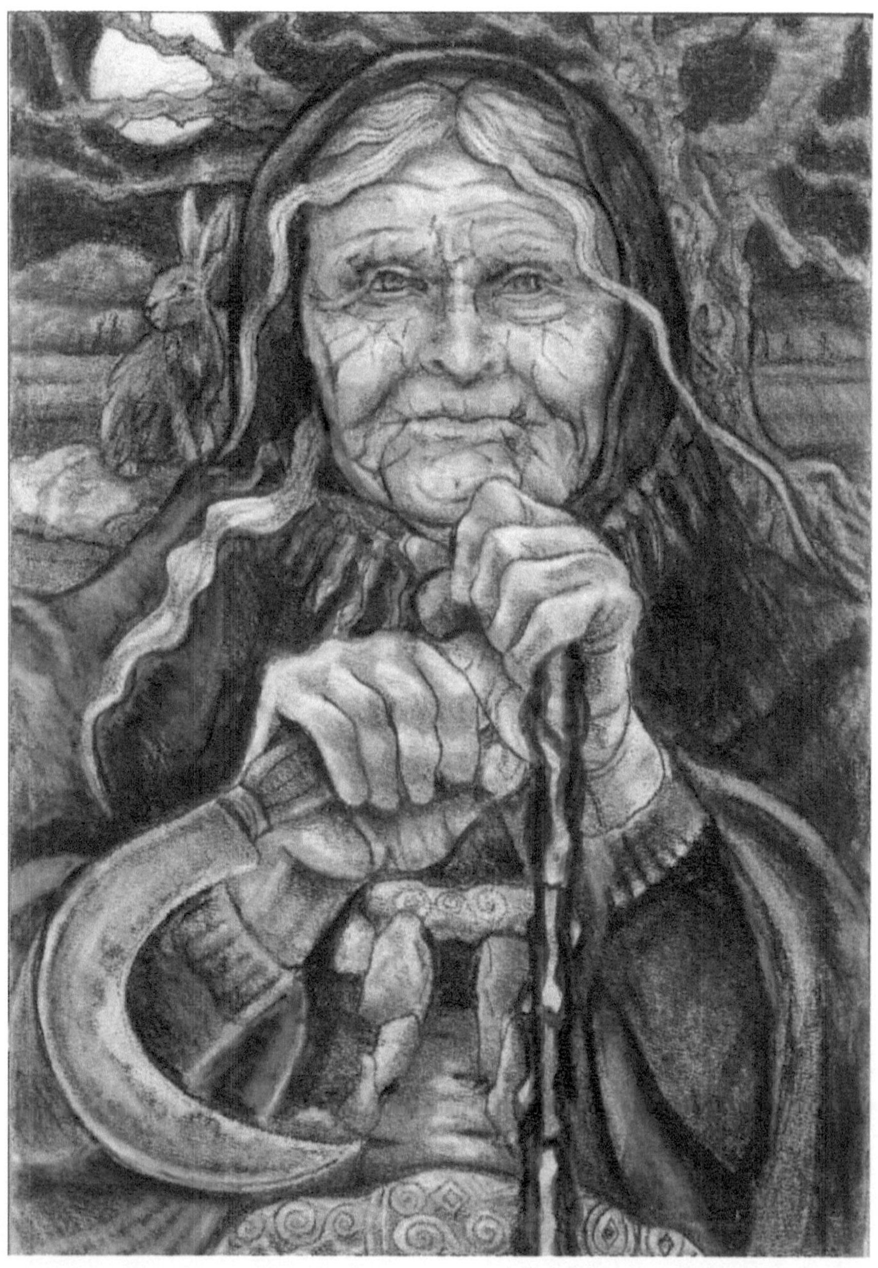

Crone Phase
Stella Webb

i am ready to move from the long last phase into another
no longer bound by the constraints of maiden or mother
my feet are wise enough to lead the way
knowing the path varies for everyone, every day
my eyes perceive more than ever before
there's much to see beyond ordinary reality's shore
my smile is knowing, but withholds judgement
the lessons of this life demand constant adjustment
my hands give and build only when they so desire
no reason to waste my time, my words, or my fire
the light and the darkness are now the same for me
fully embracing everything i can possibly be
i have collected a lifetime of lessons, both easy and hard
and i've done the soul deep work to heal my scars
i am steady, i am grounded, i am wise, i am free
the opinions of others mean absolutely nothing to me
i am loving, i am fierce, i am strong, i am wild
i can be a raging tornado or a breeze, soft and mild
i stand tall, intention in my eyes and purpose in my stride
confident i am ready to move into my Crone phase with pride

The Over-Flowing Chalice: When Red + Blue Is More Than Purple

Deborah A. Meyerriecks

My menopause journey seems to have begun in earnest in October 2017. I was 48½ years old. Fittingly, my experience seems opposite to most I've been told about. As a child (also the one who always added the "and a half" when appropriate to my age), my mother and grandmother reminded me that I was always being "contrary," as they would put it. I remember chatting with my new boyfriend and exploring the idea of a long-distance relationship with him. We met through an online mutual friend's introduction in late September 2017. Soon we were discussing the potential of my flying to his home state to meet for the first time. He wanted to make sure I was surrounded by friends and felt safe. Even though it was his home state, where we met was almost 5 hours from where he lived for me to be in proximity to those I already knew.

The hardest part for me was giving myself permission to take this time for myself. To travel cross country alone to meet someone just because I liked the way I felt when I shared time talking with him. I was doing something just because it made me happy to do it and for no other reason. This was a new experience for me. My Dynamic Duo were all grown up and adults who didn't need me there full-time. Here I was, not taking a day for myself but a week, with no long-term promises or expectations, just because I wanted to.

As someone who was motivated by acts of service, whether in my career, for my family, or in capacity as priestess to my community, this was radical. I felt my Goddess smiling in my smile as I embraced my happiness.

I had an epiphany. If we met—this new person and I—and we didn't click together in person the way we did though text and phone calls, if we weren't the other's 'person', I would be OK. I had been happy, genuinely happy, for almost 2 months. Sure, I'd be sad and more than a little bit disappointed if we didn't feel the same thing in person but that wouldn't diminish the beautiful feeling I was experiencing. I was starting to understand the part in the Charge of the Goddess where we say "all acts of love and pleasure…" I would hold on to the feeling even if I had to let go of the relationship and truly know that after all this time it was within me to find and create happiness for myself in all things. This was a powerful thought. It shouldn't have felt like a new concept but there it was, I could give myself permission to enjoy my life without expectations and without having to validate my existence because of what I could do or be for others.

I'd already let him know that while neither of us were "grossed out" by menstruation while being intimate, I never knew when I was going to cycle. Often, I would only get my cycle 3-4 times a year. Kinda like Mercury Retrograde. Unlike that little planet who keeps a sharp schedule, I never really knew when it would happen. I learned to pay attention to my physical body for announcements. A sharp but brief lower abdominal cramp generally was my 2-week warning. Swollen breasts, not unlike when they were filling with milk when my babies were ready for me to feed them, would start about a week before my flow let down. I never noticed mood swings or irritability. Just a general 'ugh' over the inconvenience of working on day 2 & 3 when my flow could saturate a super plus tampon hourly. I worked outdoors and didn't always have easy and frequent access to a bathroom.

I would mark my calendar to keep track because the common first medical question to every single woman is "what is the date of your last menstrual period?" What is your "LMP?" I'd learn over time that it was less about whether or not we might be pregnant and more so they knew which phase in the cycle of being a woman they would blame for us not feeling well.

My new boyfriend and I were looking at a visit together in November. Here it was in October. I had been an emotional wreck for a week. Highly sensitive, feeling needy for reassurance, and hating it. Who was this person? Then my flow let down. I gleefully let him know that while we were together in November, I wouldn't be able to perform any "blood magick." I bled in September and now I was bleeding again in October so there would be no way I would be ready to go through another cycle by November, right?

November came. I was hyper emotional, high strung, stressed. Well, who wouldn't be? I got on the plane. When I landed, he let me know he was not going to be able to meet me the next day as we planned due to a family emergency. I flew in a day early to get a cheap flight, planning a day of exploring on my own until he could meet up with me. Rather than a day trip to the mountains, I camped overnight and explored the next day as well. The experiences I had were a Goddess given gift. In fact, I believe I met her out on the trails. She even admonished me to drink more water. His family situation stabilized, and he drove to meet me a couple days later than expected.

When we met, I felt like a teenager hopped up on hormones being kissed for the first time. "So, this is love?" could have been the theme song in my head. Determined not to do anything to let me feel taken advantage of or vulnerable (I had already been up front with him about prior abuse and some lingering issues I had been working on within myself) he took me to our room. We talked, we cuddled, we did everything except have sex. He was very clear that this -is- love and that he was making love -with- me but I would never, ever again, be used for sex or allowed to be hurt. We discussed that if it felt right, we would share that too, over the weekend we had together.

I woke up feeling safe in his arms. Something I don't remember ever being able to do with anyone else before. I felt Goddess' presence like the soft warm glow of sunrise. I got up to use the bathroom. I doubled over with sharp, sudden cramping and down came my flow. It came without warning, leaving me nauseated and shaky for a while. I was near tears. He was kind. He helped me to the bathroom. Made sure I had what I needed and felt well enough to be on my own, then went out to get me what I needed. It felt like he returned almost immediately. He helped me back to bed, brought me a cup of decaf tea, and cleaned up the small mess on the floor.

He wouldn't take my apologies. Said I have nothing to be sorry about. Said my comfort and well-being, emotional as well as physical was what was important. When I was ready, he took me out for brunch.

What new experience was this? Not my fault? I didn't have to suck it up and pretend to be fine for the sake of someone else's comfort and expectations? I wasn't letting him down or ruining our limited time together? That my body wasn't betraying me? It was just being normal even though inconvenient for what I wanted at the time? Huh. This was indeed quite new for me. To be accepted and encouraged to accept myself as I was in the given moment and know it in no way diminished who I was nor my worthiness; this was going to take time to get used to. Why should I have needed that time? Why was this not part of my normal way of thinking and feeling? Why? It was exactly what I'd say and how I'd supported so many others through their own difficult moments.

The weekend was much like how our text and phone relationship had been for 2 months. He let me know that he saw the woman he loves. That my magick was glowing and he was just happy to be with me even if only for the weekend. He was happy that I wanted to be there with him. He didn't love me for what I used to be able to do or what I could do now. He just loved me. I remember thinking that I need to learn to love myself that way. I remember hearing Goddess whisper that she always did—and it was beyond time I did too. Now, I think that experience was one of her many gifts to me, even though it didn't feel like it at the time.

When I returned home the cycle of overwhelming emotional flux happened again. My daughter pointed it out to me. "Mom, you know how you brew the herbs into tinctures for other people? You need to do it for yourself now, too." And she was right. It was time I took the herbal care and witch-crafting I have employed for more than a few decades and care for myself. What a concept! Self-care. Looking over my calendar I noticed I began experiencing my "Monthly" or "Moon" cycle, well... monthly for 4 months while I was preparing for my 5th "Monthly" cycle in a row.

I have always been sympathetic and understanding of other women while going through their own cycles and how it made them feel emotionally, mentally, and physically. I couldn't empathize though. I long ago acknowledged that people experience different things and have different thresholds of tolerance. It just is. The world we live in needs consistency though. So there's a pill for that and you take it and hope it helps. You have to still get through your day-to-day obligations, and no one is going to slow down for you. Have a moment where you aren't managing your emotions or are getting stressed and aren't calm and clear? Well, you must be PMS'ing. It is so bad that in Emergency Medical Jargon and abbreviations, the "PMS" for Pulse, Motor, and Sensory was taken away from our use. It meant the other PMS and only the other PMS. I think it was more that juvenile behavior took over and they couldn't think past the uncomfortable. I'd like to think it's because PMS related to menstrual cycles was becoming a legitimate, cared for condition. I think that's just me wishing too much.

As I write this it has been over 4 years. In the last year it has begun changing more frequently. The way the hormone flux hits my emotional center of balance, and my physical state of well-being has been getting more... Just more. Every time I learned to manage and control it, my symptoms changed. I believe now that I'm not supposed to learn to manage and control myself. I think my Crone's lesson from Goddess is rooted in self-care and acceptance. I think my menopause journey has been to give me this last precious time to learn to let myself feel. One day my blood will no longer flow but my tears still can, and they are the releasing of emotions and feelings that are spent and meant to be experienced. Some happy, some sad. All of them in need of being released. I am learning to let them water my hopes and dreams. I am letting them lubricate my memories and my feelings and help them to flow into my present space. Life is messy. Feelings aren't meant to be tidy and organized. I don't always have to have it all together.

When I was almost 30 years old, I was facing surgery again. I had already survived cervical and ovarian cancers. This time I had another mass near my ovary and one in my uterine lining. It was a challenge to get the surgeon to agree to perform a tubal ligation. He absolutely would not perform a hysterectomy and would only do the tubal ligation with my (then) husband's permission. That I had already been pregnant 5 times with 2 healthy children surviving was beside the point. I resented needing anyone's permission to take care of myself. After a serious discussion upon seeing my scans, I was able to sign an agreement that if in the surgeon's professional opinion future pregnancies could be dangerous after removing the masses, he would do the tubal ligation. When I woke up, I learned my tubes were cut. I was relieved.

Because of where I am retired from and the work I used to do, I am in a very high-risk group for cancers. This year's pap also came with a uterine sonogram just to be safe. The results were questionable, and it was recommended I follow up with a uterine biopsy. The surgeon who performed the biopsy informed me I have an enlarged uterus which is causing abdominal distention, undue stress on my back and spinal injury, and could contribute to monthly episodes of anemia and heavy, prolonged bleeding during my cycles. His Nurse Practitioner also informed me that I could suffer extreme, heavy, and prolonged bleeding as the situation worsens with time. Even though I had discussed my intolerance for anesthesia and allergy to most pain medication and confirmed he would use neither for the biopsy procedure, this surgeon, not even knowing what my current menstrual flow was like or how I was actually feeling, recommended a hysterectomy. Why? Was it for my personal comfort, well-being, or potential safety? Was he preparing me for the what if the biopsy revealed cancer? Nope. It was because at 52 years old with 2 healthy children I'd done what I was supposed to do and my husband should not have to suffer my bloody flow interrupting his sex monthly. I was stunned. I had to hound his office for my biopsy results. Gratefully, negative.

I promised myself to find a new GYN practice, and I did. I am learning to treat myself with kindness and respect. I will take no less from my doctors. I am more than what I am to someone else. This shouldn't be a radical thought. The new GYN surgeon reviewed my scans, test results, and examined me himself. He was happy to inform me that there was absolutely nothing unusual or unhealthy with my uterus. He said the slight thickening and enlargement were only slight and directly related to the pattern of menstruation I had for 35 years plus bringing 2 larger than average babies to full term. He informed me kindly that based on our discussions and his experience, I probably have less than a year left with my monthly 'friend.' He was also firm to point out that the uterus is a powerful part of a woman and contributes much to her orgasmic pleasure even after menopause. While hormone supplement therapy could ease my symptoms, they increase my cancer risk and he recommended against them, instead suggesting a naturopath and a physical therapist. Food and movement and rest.

I am learning to take pause and rest. I no longer have to rush off to work. I can do things at my own pace and in my own time. I am still quite young but not young anymore. There are still hints of red in my sterling gray where there used to be glints of silver sparkling in my warm, multi-colored auburn hair. I can still support and care for those I love while physically being still and resting.

The lesson I have been struggling with is that I am worthy of love and that I am indeed very much loved not for what I have done or what I can do but simply because I am. I am learning to love myself. That man still holds me as his beloved and has given his heart to me time and time again. My children are adults in their own life who reach out to me to share themselves and want me to continue to share myself with them. My Tribe has assured me that regardless of what I physically can or cannot do, they value my voice, my experience, and are happy to listen when Goddess whispers Her inspiration to me and I am ready to share.

The pale pink of the red tent I never took time to realize I was invited into all along has matured to a deep, dark crimson red. Now that I have granted myself permission to enter into my red tent each month, now that I have truly spent time with myself in here, I can see it slowly starting to take on the transitioning hues as more purple is added to the red. One day, I don't know when, the red will fade enough to see it. Perhaps it isn't purple that's being added but blue.

The Red of Fire, the passionate energy of Wands and creation. It will never stop flowing. I'm learning to add more Blue of Water, with its intuitive and compassionate healing energy into my Life's Chalice.

As they blend together, the Purple of Spirit reveals itself. Spirit is really our inner self and where we truly meet with Goddess.

Perhaps my Croning is mostly about genuinely getting to know myself. Despite all the reasons I was taught not to, I really like who I am, who I've always been, and who I am becoming.

I am learning to allow myself to take up space when I feel like it.

Giving myself grace to cocoon and rest when I want to before I need to and not feel the need to make excuses for my lack of "productivity." After all, the word 'rest' is a verb. So is 'comfort." As a mother and a daughter and a medic, and a priestess, I endeavored to give comfort to others. To rest and to comfort myself should not feel like they require permission from anyone other than myself.

After offering my Chalice to nourish, heal, comfort and support others all my life, I take this time to offer it back to myself. To savor the healing water I've poured of myself time and time again. I have learned that while you can't pour from an empty cup, my cup has and always will overflow, and Goddess Bless me, there will always be enough to share. Especially with myself.

Queen of Water
Barbara O'Meara

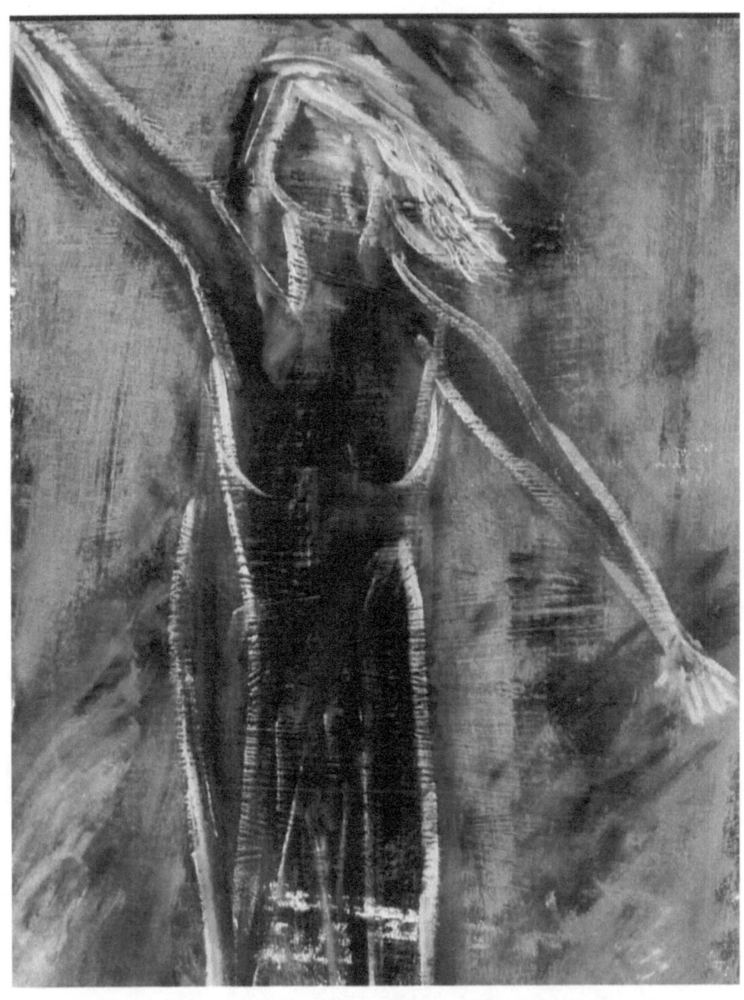

Claiming Your Crown as Crone
Barbara O'Meara

Crown of Earth

Dig deep my beloved, furrow down, make your mark, shape a trench in boggy wetlands, an indentation over arid wastelands, a track through rich dewy pastures, a rut in snow covered tundra, a ditch by coastal marshes, a fissure on molten lava fields, dig deeply through all the forgotten lands, dig from the depths of your soul, dig for your life. Claw, scratch, tear and burrow your way into a new holding space, a heart space, a perfect plot. Long nailed fingers, sharp as shards, clefting old ground, slicing through, gnarled raw hands hurling soil, casting away slapdash muck and sludge, brown turf, red clay, fine grained sand, porous limestone, solid granite, layer upon layer of strata until you reach the bedrock. You have lived it all. Churn it up using your open arms as primitive plough bones, make your descent, this is your aging rite of passage, to dig in, to dig down, descending to hollowed, all hallowed ground. Climb into your precious resting place; bury yourself in the gashed Earthen wound of your matriarchal lineage.

You are truly Queen of all lands, now you must honor your roots and claim your crown as Crone. Wear it well, this winding, binding, bulbous, tuberous contorted crown, wound tightly with the detritus and humus of all the years you have lived. Spittle seeds of hope and regeneration dribble from your scarred mouth. The feet of crows have danced on your eyes. The origin of all life dwells in your soul, all knowledge is embedded in your heart as you bed in beneath fallow ground. Here in this silent Souterrain, whether you are world-weary or well lived, you are on the cusp, between two worlds, wrapped in a protective caul of the energies of Mother Earth as she holds you in a fierce grasp.

This womanly chamber is seamed with precious veins of knowledge and wisdom which you have been mining through, all your live long days. The shapes of all things are marked out in scratching and scrapings. Whispers of keening sisters cavernously echo through in soft comfort. This is your safe place, your birthright, an honoring to commemorate you as a female elder, to bear witness to your ceremonies, rituals, rhythms and all your feminine ways from precious womb to sacred tomb.

Crown of Air

Liberate the ties that bind you, call in the winds of change. You are a visionary, a stargazer, an astral planer, element of air billows around your static form, gyrating frantically to release you from your human bondage, your foot-fastened, land-locked foundations. The feathers of your tightly shackled wings are ruffling furiously, attempting to span out, to break free. The ages of maiden and mother are behind you, now you must spread your wings, letting go of all that is mandatory, mundane, mediocre, all that no longer serves you.

Now is your time to take flight, to seek higher ground. Cast off your earthly garments, loosen your braided hair, disentangle yourself and open out your great wingspan in preparation, hold on tight, hurl yourself into the forces blowing in the vast skies. Fierce currents of air are whirling around you, sweeping you along in great gusts, as nature crafts tiny flying machines of leaves, twigs and discarded debris. Magical birds gather momentarily to admire your radiant plumage.

Soaring above the storm clouds, released from your constrictions, gazing below on all of life's trial and tribulations, you have risen above the captivity and confines of human existence. Don't look down, ever. Ecstatically elevated towards heavens reach, you are Queen of the Air. To celebrate your one true cosmic life, you must now claim your Celestial crown. Formed by flittering creatures of flight, all that is winged and airborne, enveloped in wisps of cloud, fix your fantastical fascinator onto your highly held head. Pin it on with golden quills, magnificent tail feathers, invite flocks to nestle in. Upraised to all seeing, you now defy gravity, you levitate, you are a universal aviator, piloting pioneering women through the airways to rise up, to glide with ease and to fly high transcending time and space.

Crown of Fire

There is a raging heat coursing through your body, boiling your blood to the brink of combustion, an ally against the negativity of the naysayers who would extinguish your passionate fire. Those who would douse the sparks of a mighty firebrand, quenching the flames with the dampening doubt of disillusionment. Smoke filled atmosphere from dying embers aims to darken your way, to shadow your insight, to camouflage your remarkable powers with a menacing spectral presence around the great glowing of your soul. Grab your torch and re-ignite your blazing life from the flaming pyre of the divine feminine.

Emblazon your heart, with a fierce fire starter of gathered tinder and withy sticks; with fire filled breath kiss the kindling to light up your vibrant being. You are a firestorm, brazenly dancing around a moonlit bonfire, a divine Diva of flaming crimson. Fuel the furnace of your life and hark the burning of all naming, shaming and judgmental labeling. Add with zeal all that has passed, as a propellant, to fire your engines and stoke your coals. Burn all bridges to melancholia. Gather the charcoals to fashion your Crown of Fire.

The last remaining embers of this fiery lifetime are sparking up fervently, ready to forge a new coronet, a crown of melded bronze and iron, reflecting the blood and mettle of your foremothers, those who sat in fire circles with primitive kilns, wise women, healers, weavers, potters, your tenacious ancestral womenfolk who would not be snuffed out. Now they gently gather the fragments of fired earthenware discarded over millennia and tenderly they place the pieces together, creating a monumental urn containing their warming, loving blessings and the smoldering remnants of the eternal flame to place in your hearth and in your fiery heart.

Crown of Water

Wherever there is water you are found, free floating, awash, in your element. You are a shape shifter of ocean waves, shoreline of seas, ripples of pond-water, silted sands of tidal estuaries, rocky outcrops, pebbled riverbeds, hanging fog banks over lakes and lochs, grassy hummocks, brackish water, rising steam of hot springs, melt water, rainwater, a single drop in a deep well.
Drifting gives your water body a wondrous weightlessness, it disperses all the memories of body shaming, any sense of stagnation, gloriously suspended on surface waters your breasts become buoyant, you rediscover that you are a leviathan, your unanchored form is a revelation in any aquatic source. Surging through the surf your skin smartens and shrivels in the brine; your hair surrounds you, enmeshing treasure caches from the oceans. You wade through pondweed and water lilies, shelter in safe harbors, meander through marshes and wetlands, rest a while in beds of rush and reed, bathe elegantly in glacial fjords and you drink your fill from freshwater licks and rills.

The flotsam and jetsam of your life are absorbed into the tidal ebb and flow. You have bravely swum out beyond the blue; you have reached those distant shores. Your womb space is filled to capacity with the waters of the world. You courageously navigate life's roughest seas as a skilled mariner and mistress of your own vessel. Your aging body becomes otherworldly, you are enchanted by melodic sea shanties, mesmerized by the call of sirens, and your mortal flesh falls away as you become a Selkie, wearing your spectacular seal skin with resplendent pride. You are a songstress, you hold all language, all sound, you are brimming with the rhymes of rivers and streams, the wanting wailings of dream wells, the babbling of the rivulets and brooks, forgotten sonnets incased in ice fields, lamentations lost in sunken ships, trapped and captured words in ancient sea caves.

You can restore the sweetness of all sounds, but you must intentionally inhale, gulping and swallowing, the crude curses, the grim guttural insults, the harassment of harsh words, the coarse communications, you must ingest them all, let them run through you, rinse them furiously together with fear, silence, suppression. You are the instigator of a great cleansing, washing away the filth of foul words, spitting out, purging all lies, all half-truths, thoroughly wringing out the words. The salty water of your tears dissolving all that has ever been spoken in anger against women.

The ability to self-heal is the lesson of water, to wash away, to re-hydrate and to revel in the purity of our own words and truth by the simple actions of water. Now you must claim your Crown as Queen of Water, a netted veil, phosphorous, encrusted with golden corals, floating tendrils, spiked anemones, abundantly adorned with polished mother of pearl. Now as you return to the comfort of your own skin remember to recall your Selkie self and to honor your own sacred soliloquy.

Claiming Your Crown as Crone

Grieve not for what has passed, for you have survived to claim your elemental Crown of Earth, Wind, Fire and Water. You have survived to pay tribute to the immortal Goddess energies of the Crone. You are standing strong in wisdom, earned and learned an affirmation of the privilege of reaching old age. You are no victim, you are a great survivor, a warrior woman wearing your battle wounds like a majestic cloak, and your scars are the interlacing threads woven permanently through the warp and the weft to create the very fabric of your existence.

You have placed your trust in The Cailleach as your fierce companion through times of struggle. You never accepted the faux pink life of containment or confinement nor the nonsensical trappings of a gilded cage. You held firm in your sovereignty all through your wilderness years, alone, isolated, exposed, and facing the many challenges of a wildling child, of a witchy woman. You have fought the good fight and won the right to wear your crown, now you must claim it, acknowledging the gift of your precious life, of every single drawn breath. You are representing a universal congregation of sisters, remembering those who left too soon, those who could not stay to stake their claim, those who were pushed by the wayside, and those who fell down in despair, those who were deemed disposable, and those who became disconnected, disenchanted or diseased.

Recall them all as you cast off all vestiges of perceived failings, flaws and imperfections, all wrongful conditioning, all belief that supports ideas of invalidation or insignificance, all trauma of injustice and oppression. Disregard all wrongful judgments and detach as you prepare to cast aside your temporary human form, your life must be held accountable, your longevity, a testament to your resilience, touches every woman, inspires the collective sisterhood.

Now it is time to look directly into the eyes of all women, to be a searchlight for their inner strength and gifts, to shine a spotlight on their radiant hearts, to be a guiding light leading the way. You have an immeasurable debt of gratitude to all the wise women who have gone before you, who have crossed your path, who have brightly illuminated every step of the journey for your pilgrim soul. This special female bonding, a deep connection through unconditional loving kindness, tolerance, and acceptance, is crucial to the continuation of our female lineage and to our illustrious transcendence. As a visionary you have the ability to recognize the Goddess in every girl child, in every woman, a worthy gift of insight bestowed on you, giving you supreme access to the devotion of the sacred feminine. You must cross this threshold, look beyond all physical forms of Maiden, Mother or Crone, become one with the great cosmic Mother. Your day of crowning is imminent, a magnificent coronation to mark your reign and you are rightfully, regally acknowledged, empowering you to step forward to claim your Crown as Crone.

Queen of the Air
Barbara O'Meara

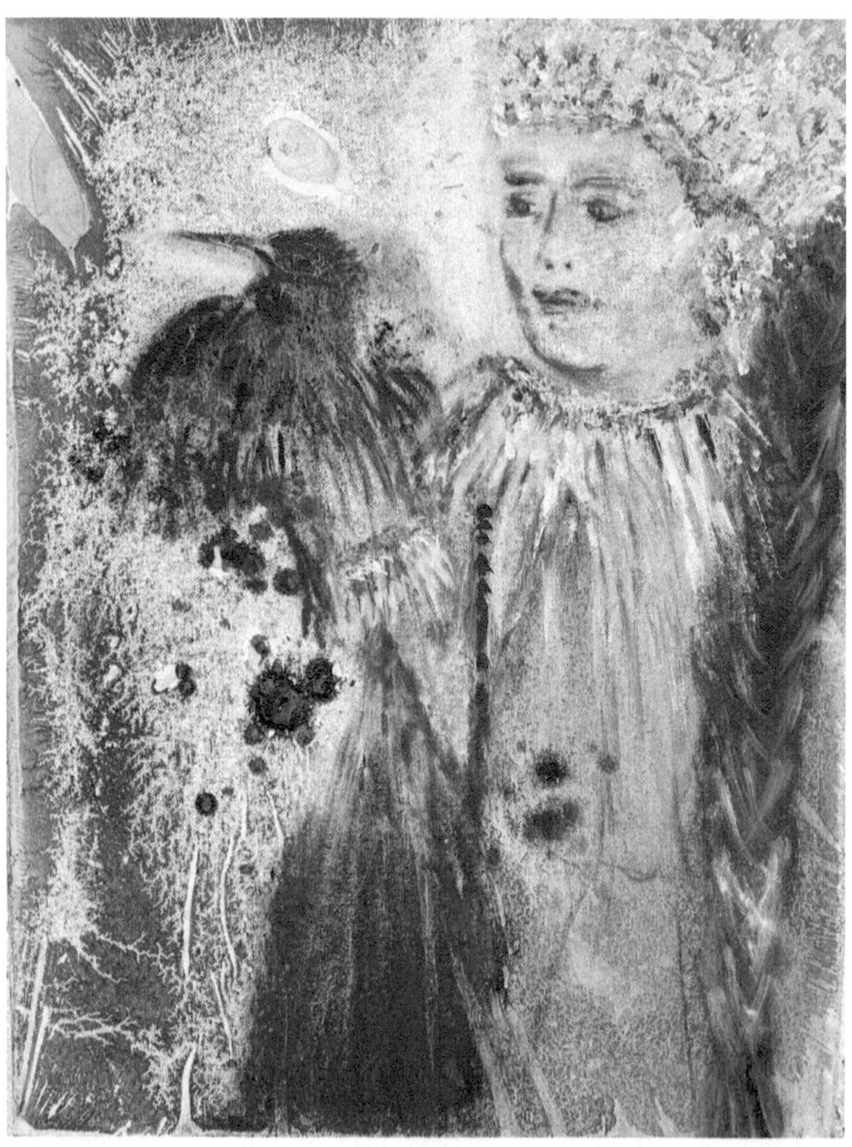

Evolution of a Crone-Queen
Sharon Smith

I hate my body, she said.
It's wrinkling... sagging.
I'm past my prime; my blood is all dried up now.
My hands: See, they are full of age spots.
My hair is turning grey.
Oh my God!
I hate my body, she said.
I'm growing old... useless... worthless.
Please don't put me in a nursing home!
Don't let me shrivel away with only
White-coated aides around me
Who really don't give a shit if I live or die.
If I get that bad, do me a favor, she begged:
Put me down, like you would a beloved pet.
I hate my body, she said.

I cried.
I saw the pain in her fading brown eyes...
Felt it in the trembling hand she laid upon my arm.
How did we get here?
How did we ever come to this?
That aging women hate their Crone bodies...
And fear for their lives as their "Golden Years" progress.
Goddamn it!
And GOD damn himself under whose male gaze
It happens every fucking day.

Because it is the male God
who has spit upon us, Who allowed his sons to
Subjugate,
Violate,
And Penetrate us. To use and abuse us.
Then throw us away when we are no longer "fertile" and
"pretty enough."
Is it any wonder we had a president
Who bragged about grabbing women's pussies?
Who called Barbie Doll women "great pieces of ass"?

I stand here today, my face wrinkled,
My body sagging, my hair turning grey...
Goddess bless it!
This... THIS is my Crone body, and I will honor it.
Despite the fact that it doesn't fit Man's "criteria for beauty."
My boobs hang to my waist.
My butt is sagging.
I have a belly roll from carrying and birthing two children.
My thighs touch in the middle.
This body has served me well...
Gotten me through hell...
Borne my scars, my pains,
My losses, my gains:
My Goddess, how fucking amazing is that?

So yeah, I refuse to go quietly into the night.
I refuse to let one more precious Sister fade away
In her post-menopausal years,
Thinking she's "not good enough"
When, by Goddess, she's EVERYTHING!

I refuse to sit idly by while Grandmothers,
Who should be honored and revered
Are left, discarded in sterile medical facilities,
Like animals at a shelter to be forgotten,
Neglected...
Abused!

I refuse! I REFUSE
To live one more day
In the shadow of a skewed and destructive system
That pits women against women
For the attention of men,
Who will toss us aside
For a younger pair of tits and a tight ass
When we begin to sag and wrinkle.

So rise up, Crone Sisters, it's time to get angry,
Time to let the Hag out of her dungeon,
Time to free the Witch from her broom closet.
Time to scream like the bloody banshees that we are!
No More! No More! No More!

We're done with the abuse and neglect,
With the stereotyping and the systemic disrespect
Of the Crone,
The Wise Woman,
The Hag,
The Witch,
The Grandmother...

Time to put on our thorn-branched Crowns
And get on down to business.
The business of reclaiming our rightful places
As Leaders,
Teachers,
Priestesses and
Seers.

Time to put away the tears and to cast aside our Fears.
Our skin may be thin, but our will is tough as tree roots
And our Wisdom, as deep as Modron's Well.
Rise up, Crone Sisters, and love your Goddess bodies!
Let no man despise you, erase or excise you.
Hug your flesh!
Shake that sagging booty!
Kiss those gnarled hands (It's your sacred duty!)
I once said it too: I hate my body…
For years I said it because I believed the lies
And for years I lived despising the advent of my
Hag hair and Crone bones,
Wishing them away with L'Oreal and Citracal
But then I awoke.

I heard the Voice of the Goddess in my dreams,
And as I got out of bed that morning,
Straightened my back and held up my graying head,
Never again, I vowed to the Great Mother,
I LOVE my body, and I'm so done with all the lies!

The words empowered me; I felt new strength surge in my bones.
Yeah, damned straight I'm a woman, aging and grey,
My Blood is dried up now,
But I'll never be ANYBODY's useless "throw-away"!

I'm a Crone-Queen! I exclaimed, and the Truth, like fire, was lit:
I deserve to be respected; so FUCK your patriarchal shit!

Sharon Smith © 2022

Queen of the Land
Barbara O'Meara

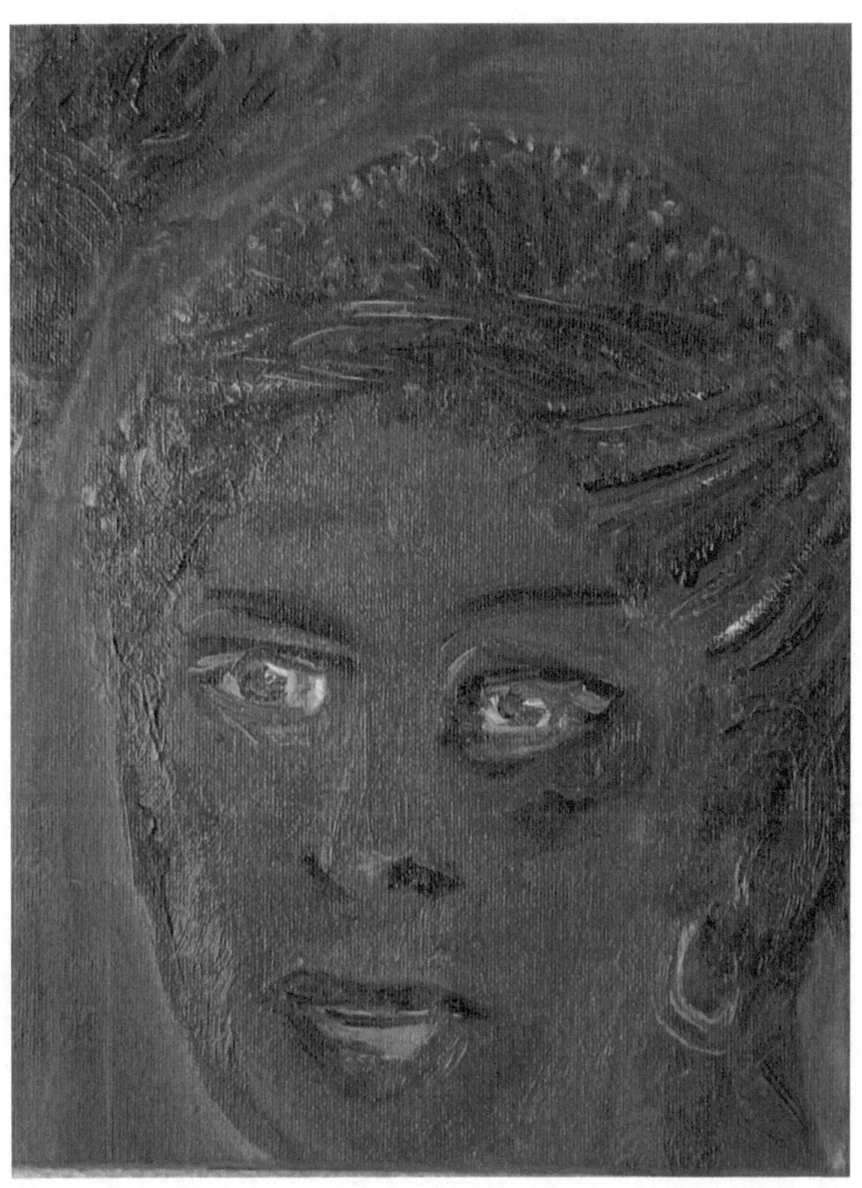

Speculations About an Old Woman on the Street

Sharon Smith

I watch her as she passes by,
small, careful steps, cane in hand,
pulling a beaten-up, two-wheeled shopping cart behind her.

She is old.
Her face deeply-lined, her eyes mere slits.
Was she trying to shut out a life of pain
and disappointment?
I could only guess…
Her hair, straggling from beneath a faded blue bandana, is
a dreary rain-sky grey.
Her hands are gnarled…
Tree root fingers grip cane and cart,
And like roots, I wonder if they ever unbend.

She wears a long coat, weather-beaten brown,
with a red patch at the hemline.
Why red? I wonder.
Maybe it's the only color she had.
Or maybe it speaks of a fire that still exists somewhere in her soul.

Is she somebody's mother… or grandmother?
At the very least she was someone's daughter.
Did she belong? Was she ever wanted?
Is she wanted now? Or has she been discarded
To live her remaining days alone… and lonely?

She pauses, looks left, right, skyward,
a slow, painful moving of her head.
chest heaving,
labored breathing.
Is she even long for this world? I wonder,
And who will miss her when she is gone?
People pass her by, on the left, on the right,
hustle-bustle scurrying mice, eyes unseeing.
She's like a Rock they instinctively navigate around,
but never take the time to admire the time-chiseled surface,
the rough-hewn angles, the darkened hollows.

They do not see her beauty…
This Crone Queen in their midst…

(This poem came to me after I saw an old woman on a busy street
in Binghamton, NY years ago. I have never forgotten her… nor the
lesson she taught me.)

Sharon Smith © 2022

The Morrigan Mask

Lauren Raine

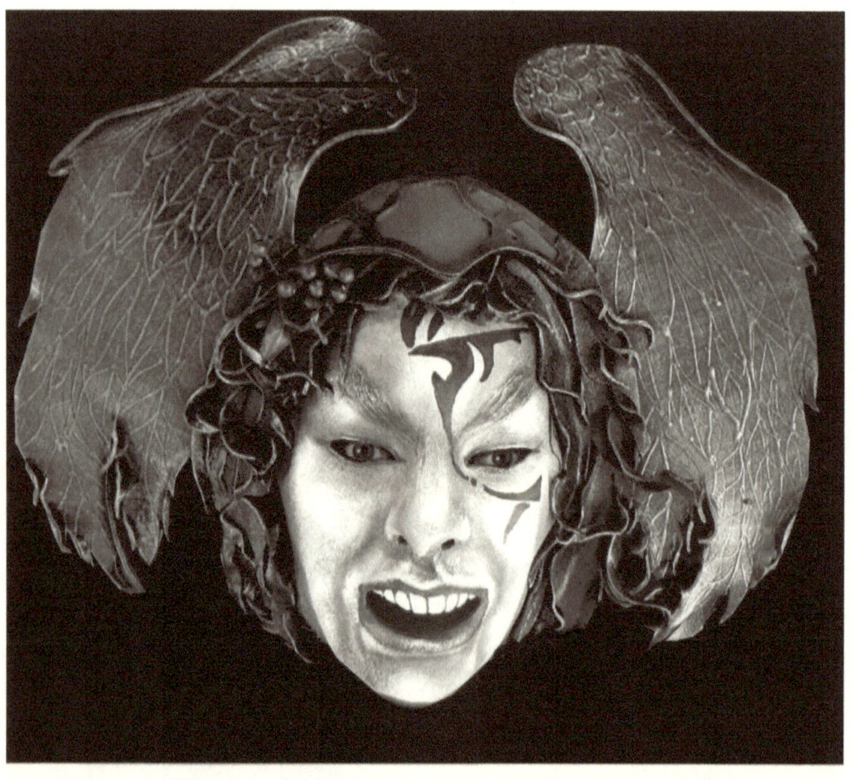

From The Masks of the Goddess Project.
masksofthegoddess.com

Phantom Queen Sovereignty: My Lifelong Journey of Initiation with Crone

Kay Louise Aldred

The Morrigan – Dark Goddess – Death Walker Crone – is the Queen of the team of Goddess archetypes I lean into and call upon within my mind, body and heart for guidance and empowerment. Her presence was activated within me during my teenage years – when moods, emotions and somatic sensations were erratic and unstable. She was the great initiatory guide who moved me through the mayhem of adolescence into womanhood.

I needed her presence in the commotion – strong, fearless and comfortable with darkness and death. Addiction and mental health challenges amongst the adults in my family and life meant I walked through shadowlands in my day-to-day life. There was no comfort externally or internally. I had no human navigating me through the traumatic swamp of my home environment and no compassionate, warm, human showing up to coregulate with me and move me through the internal landscape of chaos and increasingly mounting and stored trauma.

Inner and outer life was dark. I inhabited the underworld all day, every day.

Morrigan started the mentorship with an armouring. There was no other option. I had to become one with what I was fighting in order to conquer it. And so, the colour black called me. Black feathers. Black eye liner. Black DM boots. Long black coat. Black lace. I started to befriend the dark. She was guiding me to surrender, shapeshift into and then befriend the gloom. To become what I was resisting and feared.

Moving into the archetype of Goth – death walker – was seductive and powerful. Like Morrigan I was a walking Phantom Queen – a seer of death – predicting the unstable moods of the adults around me – feeling their trauma energies within me – choosing to harness and transmute them, rather than store them. I was making a sovereign choice. I was walking amongst the joylessness in her embodied form, and I was surviving, thriving even.

She saved my life.

Her mentorship in adulthood has supported me to develop a more sophisticated relationship with darkness, death and war – both inside and outside of me. I have noticed on many occasions that I am most comfortable in the underworld. It is a well-known place, familiar and feels safe even. I know the terrain and can navigate with my eyes shut, following an internal compass. Training as a shamanic practitioner explicitly demonstrated to me that Morrigan had activated my inner Shaman in my teenage years and that I was already skilled at shamanic journeying with her. My Shamanic Trainer called me a Spiritual Warrior and offered me the gift of black obsidian as my initiatory stone.

This obviously became exhausting.

Morrigan has shown me since that training, as I move through perimenopause, that my courage, bravery, and resilience are potent, developed and mature.

I am metamorphosising again into Crone Morrigan – the Badb – self-sufficient, highly vocal Crow.

I have a lot to say.

I don't need to be only phantom or be invisible. She has also shown that I can rest now, integrate, and sit on the throne of my sovereignty in peace. I have survived, protected my loved ones and thrived.

Beloved Crone

Andrea Redmond

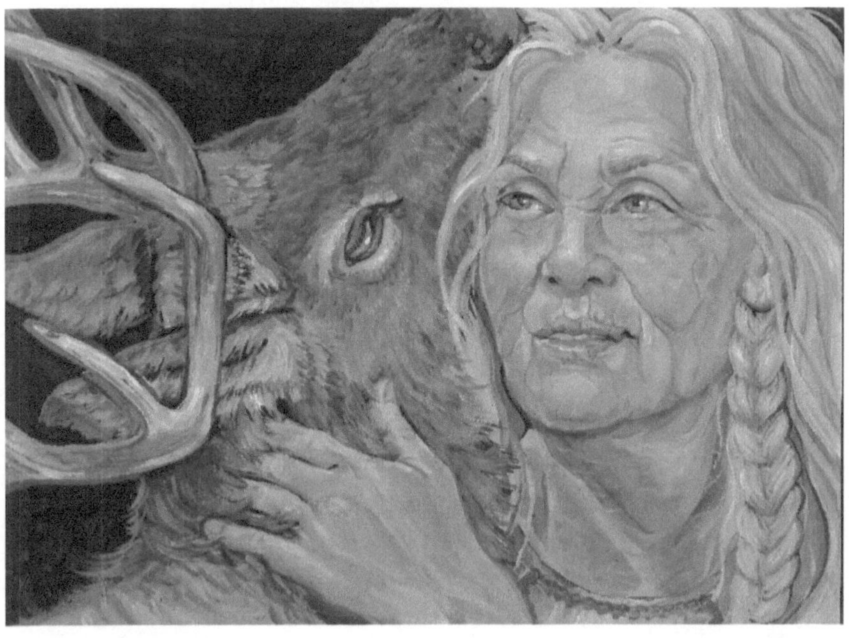

The Aging Woman

Sharon Smith

The Aging Woman... She is beautiful in so many ways.
But my heart breaks that she does not see it;
does not hear it spoken;
does not feel it returned to her so much now that her body
has changed, grown wider,
her belly a round, soft pillow for grandchildren to nestle into,
her face sagging and lined with wrinkles,
and her hair, grey as a wintry morning before the snow...

Once upon a time, she would've been revered as a queen,
when Crone was not an insult but a title of deep respect.
Once upon a time, she would've worn a crown
of oak branches, moss and acorns--a gift from the All-Mother,
because, like the oak, she has grown deep roots
over her long years and pulled up Wisdom from the Earth,
giving it out to her seedlings...

Once upon a time, they would've sung songs of praise to her
for her ample, sagging breasts that once nurtured new life,
for her Yoni in its Dark Moon phase,
that once ushered spirits into this world through its Holy Portal.

Once upon a time, she would've been cared for lovingly until she
departed this Earthly life...

But now she wonders:
will she be left in a nursing home to live out her days in loneliness,
an abandoned creature, unloved and forgotten?

What has become of Humankind, that late-blooming animal?
Deceived into thinking they are Firstborn and somehow
"greater than" all of the other creatures on planet Earth?
When they lost their connection to the All-Mother,
they lost their understanding of ALL Mothers;
And all Women have suffered, especially the Aged Ones,
Who are least appreciated and least understood.

The Aging Woman...

She can be
Apple-cheeked,
"Aunt Bea-ish",
Sassy,
Classy,
A Grand Dame,
Stylish,
Graceful...

OR

She can be
Brittle-boned,
Wiry-haired,
Stoop-shouldered,
Hunch-backed,
Gnarl-fingered,
Paper thin-skinned,
Wrinkled,
Sagging,
Sunken-eyed

BUT

She is always
Witch,
Priestess,
Healer,
Wise Woman,
Teacher,
Seer,
Edge-walker,
Grandmother.

She should be carried on a fucking gold throne
instead of stuck in a wheelchair in some dismal hallway
in a second-rate nursing home.

The Aging Woman…
She is rising up now, the Blood of her Ancestral Mothers
boiling in her veins…

The Aging Woman…
Once she led the whole world with her Wisdom and her Magick,
And, by the Goddess, she will do it again!
Come "Hell or High Water"

She will do it again!

Sharon Smith © 2022

Holy Crone
Dee Mulrooney

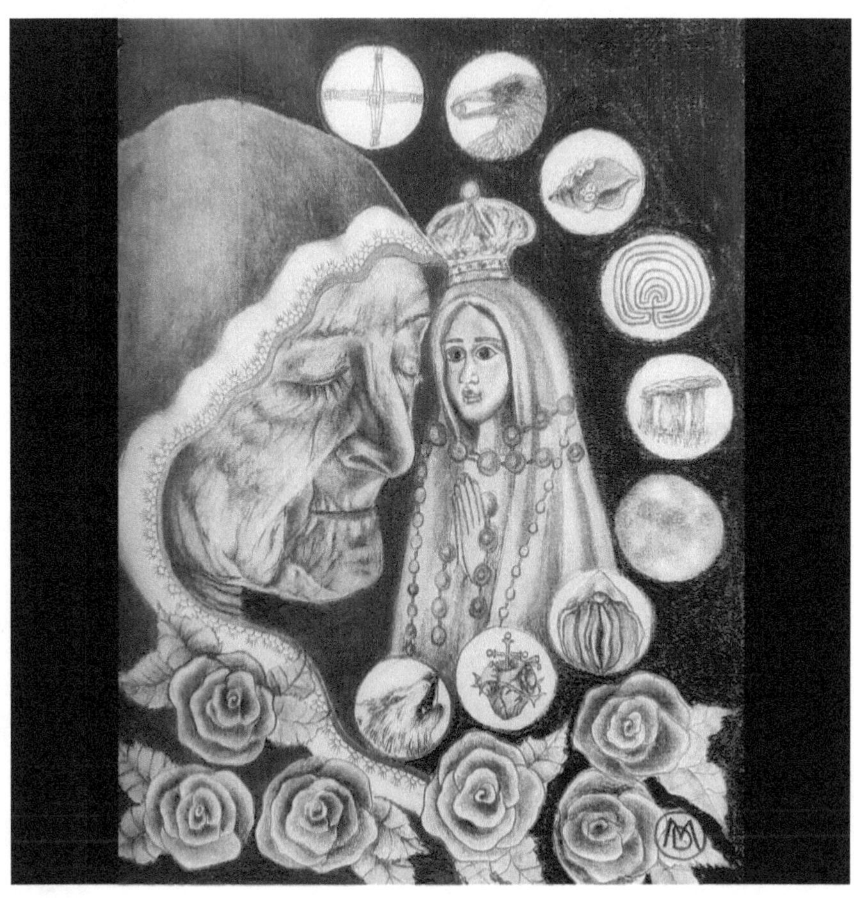

Becoming Crone
Dr Lynne Sedgmore

Introduction

As I journey through my sixties I am surrounded more and more by people dying, various illnesses and an increased awareness of my own physical ageing. The death of my mother left me, as her eldest living daughter, the oldest in my immediate family. Through the experience of watching the near death of my husband three years ago, my own relationship with death and loss directly stared me in the face. I began to accept that I have fewer years left than I have already lived.

I am being stripped of old identities that no longer serve me, however important they felt in my first half of life. I am asking important questions of myself, as a 66-year-old woman, someone who is still full of life and love; but is now keenly aware of my own mortality. Some women begin to explore Crone from their 40s, others don't feel Crone until their 60s or 70s. She will enter your life exactly when you are ready. I became a grandmother at the age of 48 but Crone didn't appear to me in a meaningful way until my 60s.

Following my 60th birthday I began to explore Goddess forms of Crone, joined a Crone circle and attended a course on Crone Empowerment. To my delight Crone poems and ceremonies began to flow through me. I learnt how to celebrate Crone through the beauty, power, wisdom and fabulous juiciness of older women.

Wise fascinating women living life to the full with all their aches and pains, as well as their good humour and high spirits. I acknowledged my experiences of loss and of facing death directly. I plunged the depths and suffering of my new Crone experiences. I discovered Crone as an important and powerful manifestation of Goddess, in the later stage of life.

I began to experience Crone from the inside out as expressed in the poem that follows:

I Am Crone

I am Crone
My black feathers rustle and soar
I have lived three score years and welcome more.
I face my future content and prepared
So many loves, lives, experiences shared
Many more to come – I thrive in my prime
Make no mistake – this is MY time
I am Crone

I am Crone
My voice crackles, keens, calls and caws
Speaking wisdom from depths of ancient years
Let me share the Goddess truth I hold dear
Chanting to release your soul from all fear
I Call in the power of kith and kin
The peace beyond all suffering
I am Crone

I am Crone
In the chambers of my black cave
I liberate women: bold, strong, wild and brave
Come and seek my face in the underworld
Allow the dark mysteries to unfurl
Swirling energies both good and unkind
Releasing all from the ties that bind
I am Crone

I am Crone

Blood, bone, black – darkness incarnate

I bring much to thrall and celebrate

Journey with me beyond all that you know

Trust in my magic and all it can show

My cauldron brews a potion bittersweet

A drink that heals and makes lives complete

I am Crone

The Crone really matters to me, as lived experience, and as archetype and Dark Goddess. She helps me to make the necessary descent of old age. She strips away all I no longer need. She holds me in times of transformation, difficult choices, death and deep transitions. Crone helps me to reduce my focus on outer appearances and to stop caring what others may think of me. As I explore and feel into myself as Crone, I become more aware of a purer, deeper wisdom, steeped in compassion, humour, courage and directness. I feel ready to express more of my authentic self and to take braver actions, and to be fierce. I am more comfortable with flaws and imperfections, both in myself, and in others. I have less energy these days and now use it more sparingly with a clearer focus and intent.

Now that I no longer menstruate, I feel free in my body as I no longer have to worry about pregnancy or hormonal fluctuations and can turn my attention to being a support and guide for those younger than myself. I don't need any limelight and am content to be in the background, encouraging and empowering others.

Crone is ignored within patriarchal and stereotypical notions of femininity. She has been distorted within the false glamour and desire for eternal youth. The dictionary definition of Crone as 'ugly old woman' is yet another expression of the stupidity of patriarchy and its repression of the glory and significance of the older woman. Many people refuse to see older women as a valuable force of powerful and potent energy. Patriarchal culture does not teach us how to see, understand or listen to Crone, yet many women are now reclaiming and celebrating Her.

I reclaim Crone as a positive, enhancing, and exciting stage of life. I refuse to be invisible or devalued and am proud to express the glory of being an older woman as an important manifestation of Goddess in my sixties, and beyond. We all have nurturing sides, and we all have fierce sides. Working with the energy and the various lessons of Crone, I am learning more about the fiercer parts of myself, and how to be more skillful, liberated, and direct. Her destructive aspects have taught me not to fear death, especially the death of my ego, and to accept, as natural, that everyone, and everything, is constantly ageing, changing and evolving. Crone is an essential part of the natural cycle of living and dying. Whatever difficult experiences I go through, I can transform. Crone holds everyone in their experiences of death, literal or symbolic, as a natural part of the cycle of life and nature. I now trust myself more deeply, and to accept that I really do know what I know, and much of that can be wisdom.

As Margaret Payerle, (2016) describes in her fascinating paper, The Croning Ceremony, within modern feminist and Goddess spirituality, Crone is reclaimed as one of the three aspects of Goddess, along with Maiden and Mother. "These three aspects also represent the three phases of a woman's life, as she moves from childhood, through puberty and her time of fertility, and then through maturity to old age. Traditionally, the third phase has always been as important and honored as the other two".

A Croning ceremony celebrates the woman who has reached this new stage of her life, honours the contributions she has made to her family, her friends, her co-workers, others, and society at large. It helps her to reframe growing older into a positive step forward, and to embrace the differences and changes. It welcomes her to the important role she will play as a wise, experienced, and valued elder.

My Ten Crone Wisdom Steps

To support and guide you on your own Crone journey I share 10 Wisdom Steps I have distilled from my own experiences of Crone, as well as my reading of Crone books, particularly the illuminating book by Jean Shinoda Bolen (2021), Crones Don't Whine. Travel well precious Sistar:

1) Being proud I am a Crone by embracing her wholeheartedly as the true gift she is through laughing, enjoying life, being juicy and passionate, not complaining, knowing what truly matters, savouring the good things and being true to my heart.

2) Being more fully in my authentic, wise and loving self without drama and with clear boundary setting.

3) Clarifying and living my true work and service for my Crone years, ensuring they nourish rather than deplete me.

4) Speaking my truth, expressing fierceness when necessary, but always being compassionate.

5) Letting go of all the hurts of the past, forgiving those that have harmed me and seeing the learning and the gifts in every part of my life.

6) Getting really clear on my energy levels, my need for rest and recuperation and finding time for myself.

7) Finding other Crones for affirmation, mutual support and understanding.

8) Choosing to be a role model for the younger generation through offering my wisdom, experience, expertise, and support.

9) Expressing my creativity in new, exciting, and challenging ways to constantly stretch myself.

10) Treating myself like the Crone Goddess I am through pampering and loving myself. Really choosing self-care and optimal health by listening to my body, eating properly, exercising each day, accepting my imperfections and the physical limitations of ageing with genuine care and appreciation.

We Crones Matter

Crones really are important in society, in so many ways. Many women are speaking out, as Crones and this Crone Initiation anthology is a fabulous initiative to celebrate and acknowledge this phase of life.

Here is another of my Crone poems from my poetry collection, *Crone Times*. This poem celebrates the gifts and talents Crones bring into the world. It is best spoken aloud with other Crones in a joyous and playful tone. I hope you enjoy it.

We Crones Matter

We are mighty Crones
Grandmothers, mothers, daughters, Sistars and Priestesses.
We hold wisdom:
Feeding the soul of the world through our learning,
mistakes and magnificence.
Dancing in joy at the beauty of the world.
We tell stories:
Stringing precious pearls on the threads of children's' lives.
Supporting the young ones in their arising and power.
We weep for all suffering – wailing out loud:
Reminding everyone why cruelty and wars must cease.
Listening to lighten the burden of heavy hearts.
We cackle wise and fierce truths:
Illuminating the powerful and the disempowered
to better the world.
Singing the songs that need to be heard.

We offer open, hugging arms to everyone:
Expressing the unstoppable force of compassion.
Loving unconditionally.
We revere our bodies as they droop, wrinkle, sag,
bend, stiffen, ache and shine:
Revealing the beauty of old age through
its seasons
and sacredness.
Walking all the times, tides, turnings and passages of life
We are mighty Crones
Grandmothers, mothers, daughters, Sistars and Priestesses.
Laughing at life.
We die with no regrets, fearless and full of grace.
So others may do the same.
Leaving memories that lighten lives and warm the cold.
For all these things, and more.
We Crones Matter.

Reflection

Having read my experiences of Crone, I wonder what Crone means to you? I offer some suggestions to reflect on Crone in your own life:

- What does Crone mean to you personally?

- How can you develop your relationship with Crone?

- What does it mean for you when you hear of Crone as one of the Dark Goddesses?

- Find and explore a book on Crone that inspires you.

- What does exploring Crone help you to learn about yourself?

- Is there anything for you about getting older, or facing death that needs to be worked on?

- How might you develop and live my 10 Crone Wisdom Steps?

- Can you find other Crones to share with and to give and gain support?

Crone Resources

I close with some resources on Crone that I have found useful and hope that my sharing encourages you to explore and express your own experience of Crone.

Lynne Sedgmore, (2019) *Crone Times:* TheaSpeaks Press

Anabel Vizcarra, *Crone, Take OFF your Veil*: Mauimama Magazine Issue 55

Jean Shinoda Bolen, (2003) Crones Don't Whine: Concentrated Wisdom for Juicy Women: Conari Press

Tiffany Curry and Seamus King, (2021) *Crone Rising*: Jazz House

Publications

Barbara G Walker, (1991) The Crone: Woman of Age, Wisdom, and Power: Bravo Ltd

Margaret Payerle, (2016) *The Croning Ceremony*, The Journal of Traditions & Beliefs: Vol. 3 , Article 11. (Online) Available at: https://engagedscholarship.csuohio.edu/jtb/vol3/iss1/11

Crone Song (2015) YouTube video, added by Touch the Earth (Online). Available at https://youtu.be/Doph_7gKkRk

Blessed Be

Cailleach
Dee Mulrooney

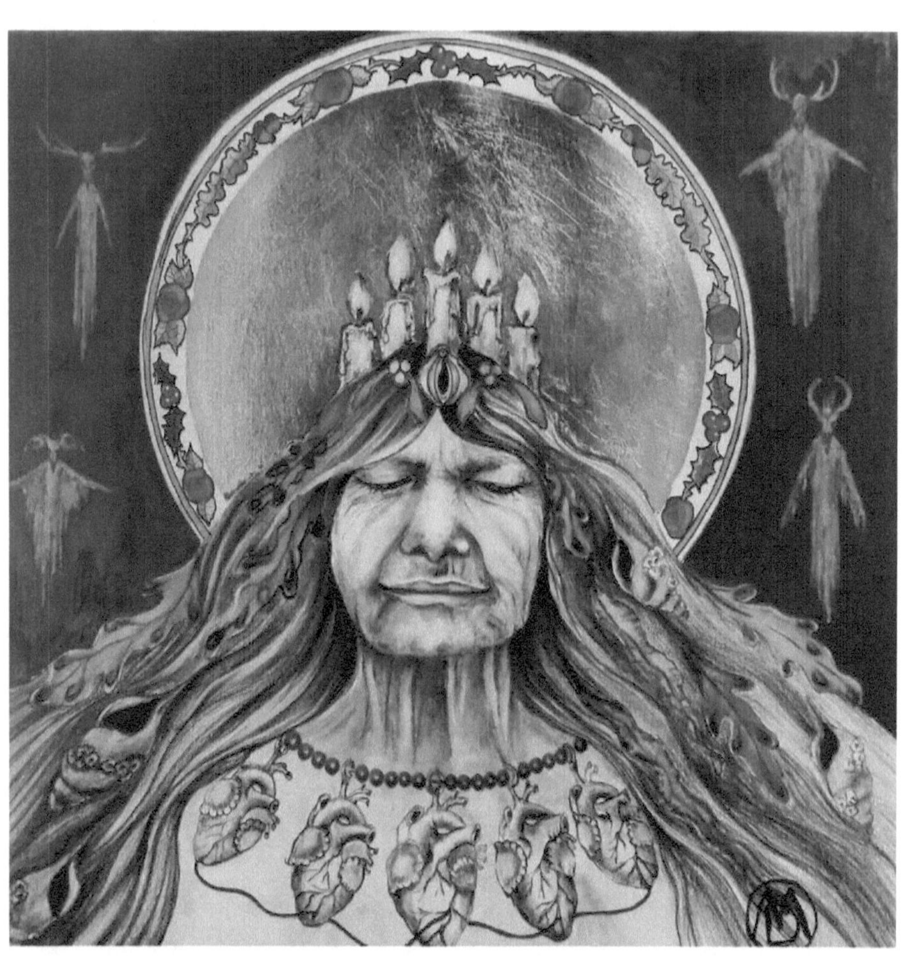

The Croning: A Ritual of American Witchcraft

Nikki Wardwell Sleath

At the time of this writing, I am 48 years old and have not yet quite physiologically exited the motherhood phase of life. I write this humbly, and with great awe and respect for my elders – for the women who have endured through life and time and continue to stay present and serve as pillars of wisdom and experience for those of us continuing on through the amazing and difficult journey that is womanhood.

I wanted to contribute, therefore, not through the personal experience of having yet successfully passed into my own crone phase, but through the sharing of a tradition that has been created in my own magickal community for the purpose of celebrating and uplifting our beloved crones. In the Society of Witchcraft and Old Magick, we have lots of special traditional rituals which the members of the priesthood are trained to administer, and one among the coming-of-age rites that we offer to our members is our Croning Ritual. Not a lot of what we do in our order is known by or available to the general public since we are a private occult order, but it is entirely possible for me to share some of the deep and important sentiment around our croning tradition here without divulging any actual oathbound material.

The whole impetus for having this ritual available to our members comes from the belief that we, as a magickal community do not want to fail where our society has failed in terms of celebrating and beautifying the aged portion of life, and fearlessly loving this stage of living that precedes death. We hoped to have a special ceremony and gathering where the aged women of our community who wished to participate would be revered and acknowledged for all of the wisdom, power, life experience, beauty and vision that they have accumulated, and that now comprises the immensely magickal being they have become.

We did succeed in creating such a ceremony a few years ago, and it was a group effort between myself and a handful of priesthood trainees at the time. Not only did we create the type of special ritual that this phase of life deserves, but we also consecrated a very special coven tool that is used in the conducting of this ritual. The croning staff is a gorgeous, human height oak staff that is wrapped in copper and obsidian wires, ornamented with keys and feathers, acorns and crystals, and various charms. It is carved with an eclectic assortment of runes and symbols and is anointed with oils. It is a special and beautiful tool that was ritually consecrated solely for use in our croning rites. The staff, on the one hand, is reminiscent of a walking stick that you might picture with popular old wizard-type characters. It can unashamedly be used as an ambulatory aid to the elder that literally helps them walk but also is a tool that conducts magickal power, especially the power that comes from deep and long-term connection to the energies of the Earth and trees around us.

The oak is a symbol of strength and longevity, and its roots are deep and wide and create a network of contacts to all kinds of DNA in the transmuting soil. The crone, like the oak, has put down many roots in this life and in so doing has been able to absorb a diverse array of wisdom, knowledge and experience from the many energies and entities with which she has come into contact. In addition to serving as a channel for drawing wisdom energy into the circle for the rite, the staff is also later laid down on the floor, serving as a symbolic threshold over which the crone will step. Just as a new couple might jump the broom in a handfasting ceremony, the crones being celebrated will purposely and consciously step over the threshold of the staff, accepting the beauty, challenges, responsibility, and respect that this upper stage of life brings.

It is a gorgeous and intense moment of stepping into the ownership of this stage of life and of feeling the transition, the contrast between the role of the mother and the role of the wise one.

In our croning ceremony, we refer to the crone as "the crown" and we honor the queenly place of importance that our elders should hold. The members often pick out a special crystal crown, circlet or headpiece of their choice with which they are literally crowned after the crossing of the staff's threshold. For members who do not favor the use of ritual crowns, a ring (which looks like a tiny crown if you think about it) may be chosen to be adorned instead. The crown or ring then becomes a reminder of the respect and royal status that comes along with embracing of cronehood and can be worn also at future coven gatherings to help keep that energy consciously afoot.

The ceremony has beautiful words that also bring us the opportunity to acknowledge many powerful Crone Goddesses such as The Cailleach, Mother Holle, Changing Woman, and Baba Yaga, as well as the crone aspects of many triple or quadruple-faced Goddesses. These energies are invited into the circle and are used to help hold the sacred power of the container that is unique to this ritual.

There is also a "Charge of the Crone" that we use which is a lovely prayer that we created and customized that sits in parallel to the well-known "Charge of the Goddess" by Doreen Valiente. The recitation of this charge is dramatic and intense and really serves to bring through the flow of the imposing truth-chills as the Crones feel themselves gaining in spiritual power. The rite also allows the participating members to have the option of changing their magickal name.

In our tradition there are only certain specific points in time where a magickal name is consecrated, namely at dedication, initiation or Croning. We realized that in acknowledging all that one has experienced by the time they are fully stepping into this phase of life, that it might also be necessary to adapt one's magickal or spiritual name to fit the differently evolved person they have now become. Priorities and worldviews can change, as can magickal talents and primary spiritual guides, and these are often things taken into consideration with the formulation of a magickal name. Also, the opportunity to formally take on a new magickal name simply helps to make this coming-of-age transition more special and to empower it uniquely according to the desired vibrations of the participant.

Lastly, and probably most importantly, our croning ritual is an opportunity for other members of the community of any age to come and witness, and to speak out in reverence of the croned participants and prop them up as we honor this life transition. We have a special altar where the celebrated crones get to bring photos from different stages of their lives, certificates or acknowledgements of various accomplishments, sentimental mementos or anything else that feels like a celebration of who they have become so far.

Surrounded by their prized photos and possessions, the other witches who have come to witness are given the opportunity to speak aloud and highlight the talents of the crones, to speak of their best qualities, the valuable traits they bring to the community and just to be able to express an outpouring of love and support for our amazing elders. In turn, the participants themselves are encouraged, if they feel so inclined, so share of their experiences in navigating menopause and having reached this stage of life. It is an opportunity to talk openly, in sacred circle and with full group support about any aspect of the process, be it challenging or amazing. We acknowledge that while some may feel the loss of menstruation, that the womb is a psychic place of creativity whether it is still in the stages of being able to physically nurture a fetus or not.

We also often speak of death as an initiation, a healing, and a final rite of passage that we may, with the right courage, look forward to in many ways. The gathering, of course, is also peppered with toasting, shared treats, lots of hugs, and of course, gifts. All in all, this croning ritual of American Witchcraft is an opportunity for a community of witches to express our respect for the crone as elder, as wise-woman, as persevering one, as sorceress, as beauty, as power, as leader, as advisor, as teacher, as psychopomp, as healer, as mentor, as empath, as experienced warrior, as grandmother, as witch, as Goddess incarnate, as death midwife and prophet, as the crowned one and as trusted friend, family member and confidante.

I hope that in sharing some concepts and components of our Croning tradition that others will also be inspired to create something similar. We can create new rituals to replace the pieces of our societal celebrations that have been long lost or neglected and yet are so important to living wholly as a community and as a human woman. To fail to celebrate and respect the elders is to remain blind to so many important facets of life, and these aspects of life and the time before death need to be embraced and loved if we are to truly live fully. A gem with any of its facets obscured does not, in fact, fully reflect all of the light that passes through it. Let us work through our fears and embrace them all.

By maiden, mother, crone and death,
By water, blood, bone and breath;
By the powers of Earth, sky and sea,
As we do your will, so shall it be!

Menopause as Rebellion
Arlene Bailey

I have come to see menopause as an act of rebellion. It's a time in a woman's life when she is finally and completely unto herself. A time when she is no longer something men want to control for she no longer bleeds nor bears children. To society she is seen as useless and becomes invisible and because society can no longer label her and put her in a box, she becomes an enigma. She also becomes free.

I finally understand why older women were treated with such disdain by society and why so many lost their lives in ancient times. If you can't label something, you can't control it and if you can't control it, it must be dangerous.

No longer do I bleed
Nor children bear
An unseen enigma
That arouses fear
But listen closely
When I say these words
I'm now more powerful
With a scream that
Pierces the veil as
I grab hold of a potency
You'll never see coming
Ignore me, berate me
But don't turn your back on me for
I'm rising into a power
You can't even imagine
Much less see or understand
You'll beg for my days of bleeding
My days of fertility
My days of youth and motherhood
For those you could control

Too late, those parts are
Transitioning and destined
To be held in the past with my old life
I am a new woman becoming
A woman who holds
Her wise blood within
And with that comes a wisdom
And power that should send
Chills through you as
I lift my skirts and let lose
A guttural scream
As the new me births

For I am free
I am Finally free!

Arlene Bailey ©2022

Selene
Kat Shaw

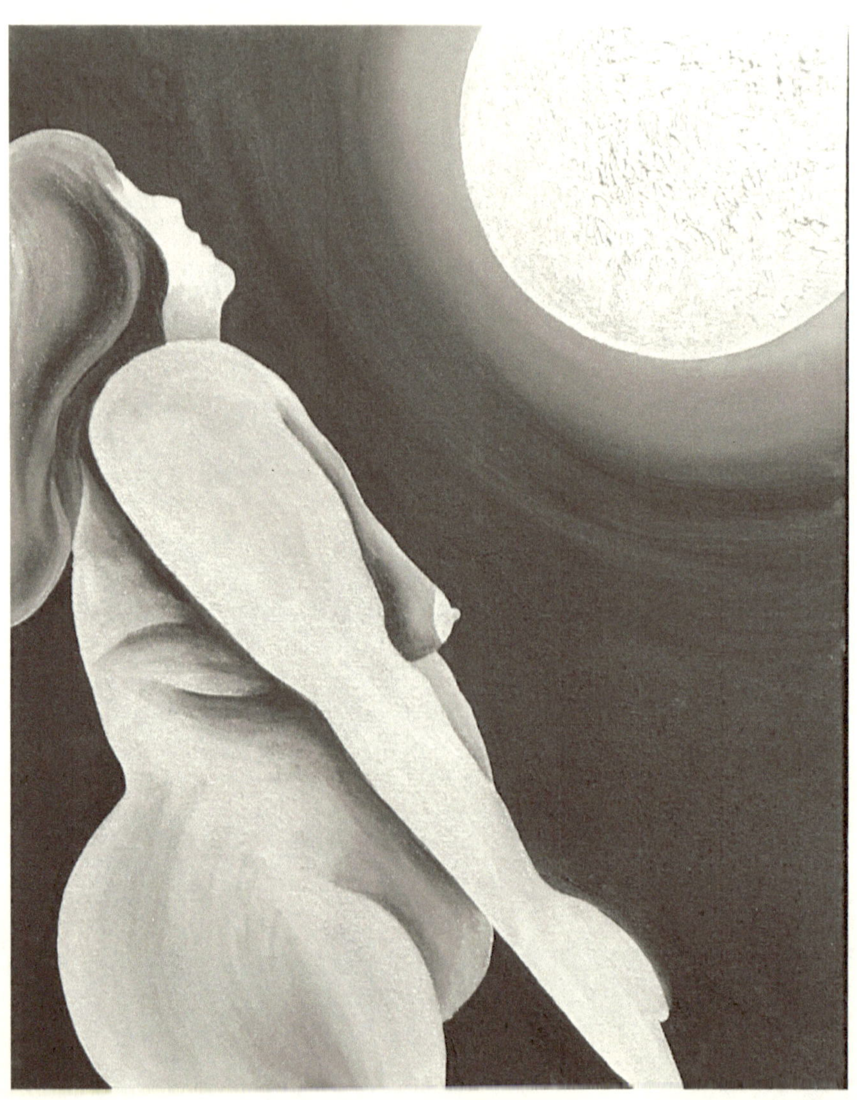

Fat is a Goddess Issue – Gateway to Khaos and Reframing the Menopause

Claire Dorey

*"Goddess is as old as the Womb of Time
and women age – get over It!"*

My name is Bee, and I bought a kaftan decorated with a neon tiger so I can waft about wearing power symbols. Sunsuna, the Great Goddess says, "You have built your temple, tamed the lion and claimed your right to the throne."

Menos Pausis punched me in the cochlea! One morning I woke up deaf and although I enjoy the freedom of silence, part of me is worried, "What if this deafness is permanent?"

Over the next few months flashes of feverish lumps and bumps, helter skelter hormones, inflammation and muscle aches rip through me like wildfire. Goodbye balance, serenity and inner peace. Hello, humiliating sweating and turning down invites.

Goodbye hip bones. Hello weight gain and acne.

I use the Greek term *Menos Pausis*, which can be translated as, 'ceasing to be present' and 'starting to perish,' to show how ghosts of ancient patriarchal language shadow women. These ghosts box in our thoughts. The ancient Greeks, whose mythology legitimised rape, believed the male body was superior because men age slower – which I dispute. A flourishing female body was a pregnant one and a female body, post breeding age, was redundant. It's time to dismantle this deluded 'clinging to' archaic values and question how doing so still denigrates women. We should not be defined by our reproductive status.

The Greeks and Romans colonised their Goddesses in the same way they colonised women, farm animals, and land. Goddess asks us to ditch the archaic term menopause and replace it with the liberating term 'Lunar Gateway' because this is our chrysalis, our rite of passage – a time of metamorphosis – a cleansing, transformative, enlightening, primordial voyage.

Free from its mental bondage, patriarchy fears the innate wisdom of the older woman, claiming we are displeasing, wicked, and serpentine. We live in hostile times. Before patriarchy was even a concept, older women were revered as symbols of wisdom and abundance.

We 'Lunar Gateway Women' can walk our sacred journey, hand in hand with a plethora of Goddesses, who are there to nourish, protect and empower. Goddesses are veterans, existing since the 'womb of time.' Patriarchy has only existed for a nano second, an irascible toddler, getting things wrong, destroying its own mother, the Tellus Mater, Mother Earth. How stupid is that? We must not let petty, petulant patriarchy intimidate and shame us at this sensitive time. We need to incubate in peace. Reaching back into the past, to find our prehistoric Goddess ancestors, we can harness their raw, primordial power and emerge through the "Lunar Gateway' – like butterflies – revilatised!

We sit in a sacred healing circle asking Goddess for advice about navigating nature's turbulent and liberating journey. As Goddess speaks, I relax and my hearing returns.

"Bee, all Goddesses have messages in their iconography that can empower the 'Gateway Woman.'" explains the Great Goddess Sunsuna. "BTW I pass my wisdom through the female line."

"I built the mother and daughter Ggantija temples, in Gozo, lugging the hefty boulders, on my shoulders, whilst carrying my daughter on my hip!" Says Sunsuna.

These neolithic, matrilineal temples, with their voluptuous labial lobes and vulva-esque entrance, embody Female Power. In ariel view, they emulate the curves of the Goddess. I've been told this is tenuous, but I can't help thinking the temples are similar in shape to the Akoko Nan – African symbol of parental protection.

Sunsuna says, "I built my temple in my own image and now I will sit in it."

The voluptuous seated icons, found in her temples, show she did this!

The cliche is true. Our bodies are our temples!

"I have lugged life's boulders and absorbed sooo many toxins." I say.

The thought of off-loading my 'back breaking burdens', cutting down on commitments and languishing in my temple, makes me feel free.

"The 'Gateway' is the time to give your store of emotional toxins to the therapist." Advises Sunsuna.

"Purge! Purge! Purge!"

It hits me that I should address suppressed trauma, or my body will erupt like a volcano!

Sunsuna ate a vegetarian diet of broad beans and honey.

"Don't consume animal suffering whilst off-loading your own suffering." She implores.

Broad beans are sacred food, regenerative seeds, symbols of death and rebirth. Honey is divine, symbolising immortality and female fertility, not just reproductive fertility – intellectual fertility!

Gozo's sister island, Malta, 'honey island' – mel is Latin for honey – is famous for it.

Was Sunsuna's honey 'mad hallucinogenic honey' – made from Ericaceous pollen?

"Did you have a 'special way' of 'seeing'? Were you drunk on honey, dreams, and visions?" I ask.

"I'll never tell! But opening the mind is crucial for you now!"

Another bootylicious Goddess, drunk on dreams and visions, is the Sleeping Lady of the Hypogeum of Hal Saflieni, in Malta, who heals in the underground temple echo chamber by incubating dreams.

She says restorative sleep is important for 'Gateway Women.'

"Use the liminal spaces, between deep sleep and waking, for self-hypnosis and to access your inner intuition and divine creative wisdom."

Fat is a Goddess issue. It represents nature's cornucopia. In the past, the older, fleshed out, Earth Mother was prized as a symbol of abundance and a successful society. Today, patriarchy fat shames us and demands we conform to a standardised body shape, which is grueling for the 'Gateway Woman' as her natural shape 'relaxes.

Mother Earth says, "Do not let them shame you with biblical accusations of gluttony and sloth. Not all women are thin. The most successful women, in all of history, were big women – so get over it!"

Icons show us that Sunsuna, the Sleeping Lady and the Seated Woman of Çatalhöyük were buxom!

"Yes!" Says spherical, Mother Earth, Gaia, "This ample hipped, Creatrix Protector Goddess, languished between two lions, whilst birthing generations and IDEAS!"

As our body rhythms change, so do our sleep patterns.

"If you are suffering insomnia or night anxiety, take this precious opportunity to spend time with me." whispers Nyx, omnipotent Dark Mother; conduit to Dark Matter; intuitive wisdom; primordial sexual energy and dreams. She is Goddess of the deep night and daughter of Chaos (Khaos) – the cosmic void of consciousness and force of creation.

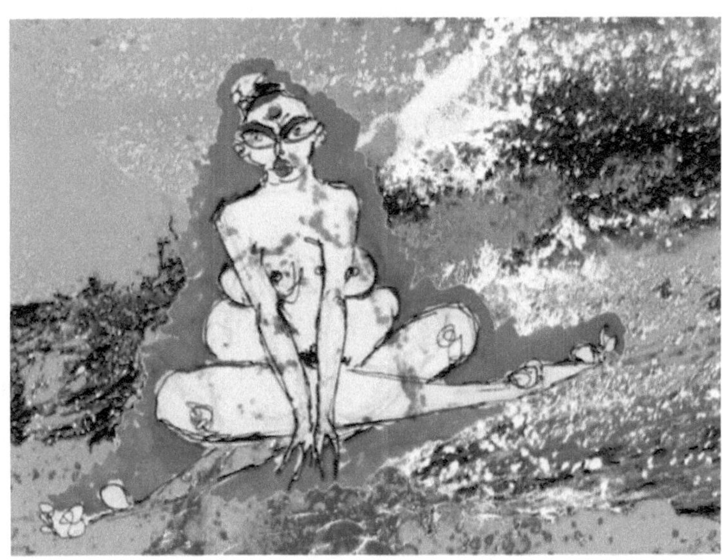

Painting by Claire Dorey

Wow! I had never considered that night sweats might be the cosmos calling!

"I will cloak you in velvety darkness so you can claim the night as your own."

"I dreamt all men and gods, including Zeus, are afraid of you?" I say.

"Chaos is female space. The cosmos is female. Women step into their power when darkness veils and moonlight purifies. We are all daughters of the moon."

"Pull a chair up to the window and take a moon bath." Purrs Nyx.

"Plant a night garden dreamscape. Evening Primrose, Night-blooming Jasmine, Nicotiana and Moonflower will pulse fragrance after dark."

Now is the time for planting the seeds of personal transformation.

The luminescent Moon Goddess Hecate was my inspiration for renaming 'Menos Pausis' the 'Lunar Gateway' because she holds the key to sacred knowledge. Maiden, mother and crone, She embodies all stages of a woman's life, transcending all realms, past present and future, darting between sea and sky, diving into the underworld.

"Sometimes I feel like hiding in the shadows." I tell Hecate. "Be kind to yourself at this sensitive time." She replies.

"Just as the moon purifies each month, we can use the 'Lunar Gateway' to purge life's accumulated toxins."

"And gain clarity!"

"Use the moon to invoke Selene, Artemis and Diana." Says Hecate.

"We all need mentoring during the 'dark night of the soul', which is how passing through the 'Lunar Gateway' can feel."

"If you do go underground to pupate, I have a tool kit of regenerative serpents, boundaries, baying hounds and feline familiars to protect you!"

Standing at the crossroads, Hecate holds a flame to light the way. "Which path do I take?" I ask.

"All paths are valid." She replies. "Step into your wisdom."

Hecate's stash of illusion slashing daggers, magic herbs, potent spells and mystifying moon rituals bring our own strengths into focus – strengths we often forget.

"We carry the imprint of a lineage of overlooked female scientists and priestesses: Maria Hebraea, Cleopatra the Alchemist, Medera and Taphnutia… and many, many more! The Witches of Thessaly were actually astrologers and astronomers! My own mother Asteria, Goddess of cascading stars, was an astrologer and magician."

I'm staring at the heavens, envisioning these high-achieving sky gazers, when Carthaginian White Goddess Tanit moves into my eyeline.

Tanit often takes the form of an ankh, reaching for the stars.

"You are literally a Female Power symbol!" I say.

"The Tyet and Venus Cross are also symbols of Female Power!" She replies. "Wear one as an amulet!"

"When you raise your hand, I can't help thinking of the Abhaya mudrā – the sacred hand gesture of fearlessness." I say.

"It's true I am a warrior." Says Tanit. "A warrior, on the side of women!"

Tanit's legacy lives on. She is still revered as a Goddess of Dance and guru for women, on Ibiza, Mediterranean island of lime white and salt; 'peace and love' and 60's hippy, anti-militarist culture.

Ibiza's cosmic dance culture is still going strong.

"Let go. Feel free. You are never too old to dance at full moon beach parties and sway to the rhythm of the universe." She says.

"Listen to the cosmic vibration and let trance become your mantra."

What a moment to have a hot flush! I was feeling liberated, when this crippling, straight jacket of infernal heat hits me. I am 'victim to hormones'!

Bawdy, crone Baubo, Goddess of the darker side of girly humour, sashays over.

"Bee, the best healing is a good old belly laugh!" She says.

Baubo's face sits in the blubber of her bulbous belly and her chin rests on her vulva. She embodies the female spirit and divine female sexual power – Shakti, in all its forms, including lewd jokes! I can't help sniggering at how comical she looks!

"When your body lets you down, laughter is the best medicine!"

"Choose natural environments with plenty of ventilation!" Advises Aura, Goddess of the cool, fresh breeze. "Reject anything fake. Go outside. Dig in the Earth. Connect with Mother Nature!"

"Try wild water swimming." Suggests The Morrigan. "I live to splash in cool lakes and rivers!"

"Carry a beautiful painted fan" Advises Isis, cooling me with her kaleidoscopic wings.

"What about fashion?" I ask, admiring her dazzling solar headdress.

I'm a firm believer that when you love what you wear you be in 'flow' and not feel self-conscious.

"More is more darling! Be bold! Wear colour, pattern and bangles." She purrs.

"BTW just because I enjoy fashion it doesn't mean I can't build civilisations!"

Isis loves her gold, lapis and red jasper.

"Wear rich, healing colours and intoxicating scents!" She coos.

"My favourites are amber oil, sandalwood, cinnamon, and orange! Seek your 'happy' fragrance and waft as you walk!"

"Bee your kaftan is lovely!" Shrieks Durga, the Hindu Goddess who is actually riding Her tiger!

"Why did you choose it?"

The tiger on my kaftan and Durga's tiger come face to face! How utterly embarrassing!

"Um! It makes me feel wild and wonderful!" I stammer.

Durga, the 'invincible,' more potent than any male Hindu divinity, is a Shakti Goddess – the divine, female cosmic force of creation!

"Your 'tiger' shows you are tuning in to your intuition and creativity!" She says.

The 'Gateway' is the time women can peel back their protective layers to reveal their imagination. Creative wisdom and artistry are powerful forces! They will free you!

"Can I have the last word please?" Asks Medusa, Her hair, a writhing halo of snakes.

"Don't let them cut your hair." She implores. "Patriarchy demonised my hair and they'll try to demonise yours. Remember 'chic' is just another word for 'conform.' Be proud of your greys! Plait it, bun it, pin it – don't bin it! Dye it pink if you want, but don't let them back you into a corner with a pair of scissors!"

Cherish yourself as you are. Be proud of what makes you! NOW is your time to bloom!

References:

Menopause in the Ancient Greek World. Kristen M. Gentile (Ohio State University).

"Goddess Tanit Ibiza – Searching for the Goddess," Michele Knight (YouTube).

"Symbolic meaning and use of broad beans in traditional foods of the Mediterranean Basin and the Middle East" by Antonella Pasqualone Ali Abdallah and Carmine Summo – *Journal of Ethnic Foods.*

Ġgantija Temples – Visit Gozo. Ancient Religion of the Great Sunsuna Goddess by C Deguara MA PHD. Ggantija – The Giant's Tower In Gozo by Antione P Borg – *The Unexpected Traveller.*

Medusa Self-Portrait
Liliana Kleiner

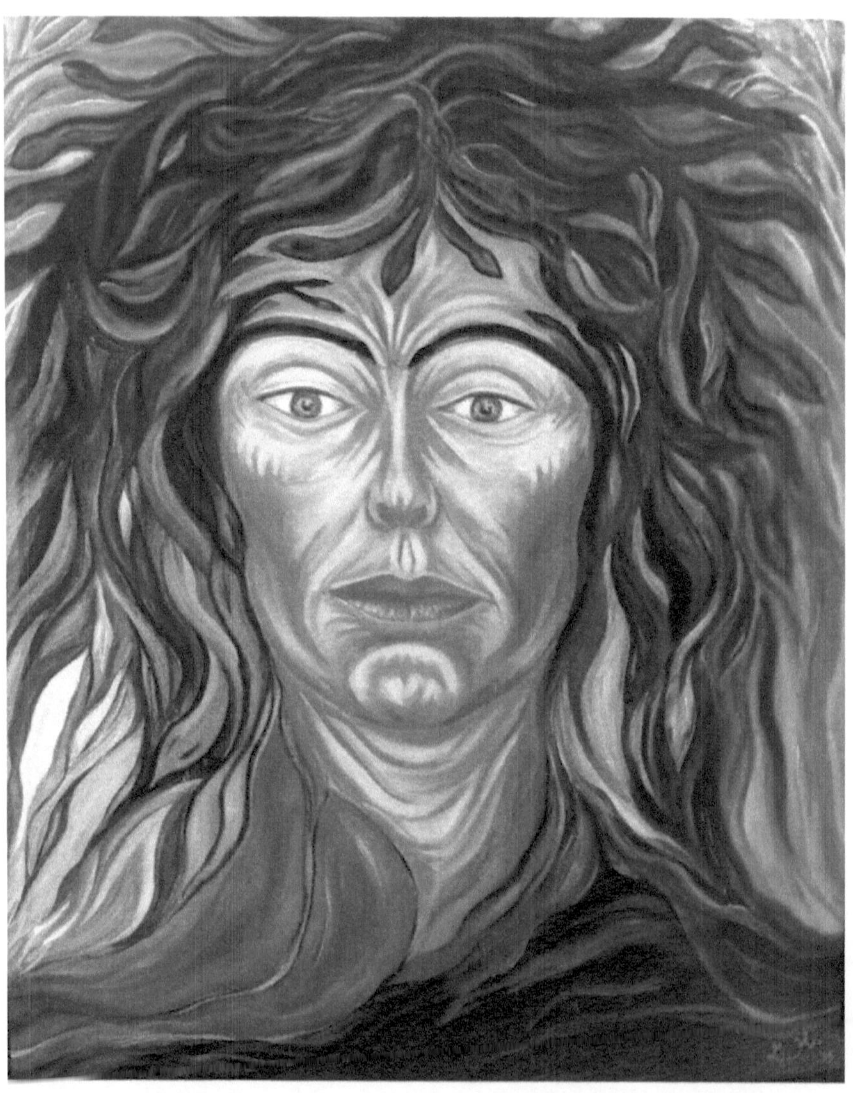

Unnatural Medical Menopause at 29: How Women's Ways of Ritual and Story Allowed Me to Reclaim this Right of Passage from the Rape of Modern Medicine

Arlene Bailey

The Ritual

As we each entered the womb space – a round, darkened tent covered inside and out with women's menstrual art – the drums beat louder and louder and faster and faster. I could hear the women inside chanting... I AM A BLEEDING WOMAN... I AM A BLEEDING WOMAN... I AM A BLEEDING WOMAN on and on and on.

In the darkness with only candles burning on altars, each woman made her way to that particular place that drew her in as she joined the others in chant. No other words were spoken. This was a sacred space and time and we'd come here to engage in holy ritual honoring and celebrating our first blood and, for some, the time of the last bleeding.

Slowly, one by one, each woman – clothed only in a dress or skirt and top – took her turn at the dark moon altar as the chant grew louder and with a feral energy of one who knows what it is to bleed.

As each woman came to this altar, she spread her legs on each side of a huge bowl formed out of Mother Earth and fired with ancient symbols representing Goddess and Woman's ways, especially those of the Dark Moon and woman's Moon Blood. As the drumming and chanting grew more intense, each woman who felt called entered the realm of the Dark Moon and lifted her garment above her waist. A Priestess then painted her abdomen and yoni allowing the liquid – made from natural clay pigments to create the color of blood – to flow down each leg dripping into the bowl as though it was a pool of her blood. Then each woman's moon blood was scooped up and put in a dark bottle and given to her as a symbol of remembering and re-membering.

I remember feeling completely inadequate, a trespasser even on holy ground that no longer belonged to me as I stood there thinking "but I have nothing inside of me left that is of a woman's cycle". No matter, for the ritual allowed for that and before the Priestess began putting the blood on my abdomen and yoni, two other Priestesses wrapped my womb space in soft flesh-tone flannel... layers and layers to represent what would be sluffing off as I bled. Then the painting began on my abdomen as each layer of flannel was covered with more and more moon blood and with each droplet that began to drip down my yoni and my legs, a layer of the now blood red flannel was removed mimicking menstrual layers sluffing off.

I remember tears flowing and flowing, unable to stop crying for all I'd lost and what I had just gained. For days my memory flashed between the time of this ritual and 1962 when my first blood came.

The Remembering

It was 1962 and at age 9 and in the fourth grade, I began my first blood. All I had been told about this time in the life of a female came from the local Health Unit. Their basic message was at a certain age, females would begin to bleed each month from their vagina. This was normal and was the body's way of getting rid of "bad" blood that it no longer needed. My mother told me nothing until I began to bleed and then it was only to ensure that my menstrual pads were well wrapped and hidden at the bottom of the trash can so my father and brother would not see them and to be sure I washed well so I wouldn't smell.

As I got older, with each month my "periods" became worse. While most of my friends bled about 3 days with little pain, I bled for seven full days with huge clots forcing me to change my pad (there were NO tampons in the 1960's) every hour or so. This went on through high school and college and into my marriage. With each year my cycle worsened and, at the age of 28, I was told I had severe endometriosis and needed a hysterectomy... a "total" one where they would take not only my uterus but my ovaries as well.

I married at 20 and, while my husband and I were not sure we wanted children, the idea that agreeing to this surgery would make that impossible haunted us both. I so desperately wanted to talk to the women in my life, but my grandmother had died when I was 18 and my Mother died four days after my 26th birthday in 1979.

Finally, in 1982 I gave in as I'd reached that place of having maybe one good week out of every month and being in pain and agony the other three. The horrors of endometriosis were barely known at this time, and I certainly had not yet discovered women's ways, women's natural medicines or the rituals around my bleeding.

Every person I saw and talked to was male.

After surgery, as I was waking up my doctor came in and informed me that they had also removed my appendix as "I didn't really need it." I remember thinking... well, actually I couldn't think. I was just in shock from having so many parts removed and trashed as though they were yesterday's leftovers. I remember feeling like a leftover and wondering how I was to live without those "unnecessary" parts.

I was in the hospital for three days and then sent home, but not before being told I was being given a prescription for a hormone patch that would help IF I had any side effects from the surgery. They (male doctors) said I "might" experience some "mild" hormonal changes and the medicine would help. Again, I wasn't asked what I wanted, only told what I needed to do. Never was I asked if I understood or if I had questions and I definitely was not told that the medicine – known as Premarin – was horse urine from pregnant mares. I barely understood what had happened and had no questions at that time for I was in shock.

I went home and one week later, I remember forcing myself to go sit in my garden and weed. I was so proud of myself for getting up out of bed, going outside and weeding. Granted I had to do it sitting on the ground, but I did it. I repeated this every day until I was back to "normal". Well normal until the hot flashes and night sweats began – you know, the "mild" hormonal changes I was told might happen. I would realize years later what a load of crap I'd been fed by male gynecologists (few to no female ones at that time) who had absolutely no understanding of women's bodies and processes or what this clinical maiming does to a woman's psyche.

At 29 years of age, I was told I had no ovaries, no fallopian tubes, no womb, and no appendix (that was gratis according to my doctor). I would never again bleed and didn't have to worry about getting pregnant. They offered that last part as though I'd just won the lottery! What I wasn't told was that I'd enter surgical menopause within three weeks of the surgery, be given a medicine made from a mare's urine, and have to wear it the rest of my life or risk the symptoms returning. I also was not told I'd feel an emptiness that offered no words of explanation.

So, being the product of modern medicine's conditioning and brain washing, I went through my 30's, 40's and into my 50's wearing that damn patch 24/7 and listening to women who did still bleed speak of how "lucky" I was. Several times I tried to quit, but the hot flashes, night sweats and crazy feelings and tears would come back, each time stronger and more intense. So I'd give up and go back to the patch. With each year, more and more I mourned the loss of my body's natural functions and those parts and rituals that made me a woman.

The Re-Membering

In my late 40's I discovered the New Age section in bookstores and began reading books on witchcraft, Goddess traditions and women's spirituality. My mind began expanding beyond the male conditioning of my youth and the questions poured through my psyche. I began to feel violated and angry that "my parts" were tossed away as though they were evil and useless for anything but creating and growing another human. I would not rest until I found some understanding! About this time, we moved to North Carolina and I discovered a haven of women fluent in the ways of nature and women's cycles and ancient ways and traditions. So, I began studying with both an herbalist and a woman teaching the priestess arts along with what she called Herstory.

I learned about menopause – a word I'm not sure I really knew the meaning of or at least knew very little of what it was. My mother never spoke about hers – if she even reached menopause as I remember she too had a hysterectomy in her late 40's or maybe very early 50's. She died at 54 so I was never able to ask her about her experience – or if she even began menopause before the surgery happened. I felt so lost and so empty. I felt as though I was not a "complete" woman. As my friends began menopause, I was actually jealous. I was still wearing that stupid patch and still felt empty within.

As I learned more about herbs – especially women's herbs AND learned more about ancient and traditional women's ways – like red tents, celebrating a girl's first blood, celebrating a woman's cessation of bleeding (what the medical community called menopause), I could feel a hunger growing for more answers and something I could not yet name, but later would learn was ritual. I read every book I could find on women's natural health and cycles and what happens to a woman when an "unnatural" event stops the flow of our natural cycles and throws us into premature menopause. There were not that many resources, but through the Priestess lineage I was now apprenticing with and with the study of natural plant medicine, I began to gain some understanding.

One of the biggest aha's! came when I realized the "why" of why right after surgery I so desperately needed to be out in my garden… why I needed to sit in Mother Earth's lap with my hands in the dirt (her body) and work with her children (the plants). It all suddenly made total sense! I was desperately trying to reconnect to my body through the touch of Mama Gaia and ancient women's ways. I was desperate to reach back through layers and layers of that dirt, through hundreds and hundreds of years to reclaim women's ways. I was desperately trying to feel the energy of the Mother, the energy of woman, in the space that was now a void rid of all of woman's natural cycles.

In 2007, having finished both my herbal and priestess apprenticeships, I began teaching plant medicine and began facilitating women's circles. As we talked about women's ways, women's cycles and the medicine that Mama Gaia had given us I began to feel more and more uncomfortable with the Premarin patch I still wore. I grew more and more angry with patriarchy's mare's urine patch and what it does to horses and women. I thought, "HOW can I be an advocate for women's natural ways and cycles, plus Nature's medicine and Her ways as long as this damn patch is part of me?" I remember ripping it off that very night and throwing away every other patch I had.

In retrospect that was pretty stupid because within days I was thrown into full blown menopause! I should have tapered down and slowly made the transition, but I'd had all of Patriarchy's control of my body that I could stand. I was now about 57 and I fucking didn't care. I knew my menopause would not be like other women – well most other women – but at least it would be more natural and I'd get to experience what I'd only heard about. Knowing this somehow made me feel more like a woman than I'd felt since my I was 29 and pre-hysterectomy.

Ooy! It's a good thing I had no idea what I was stepping into!! Hot flashes and memory loss, night sweats and more changes than I could count. My body was like "what the hell have you done to me?" My response... "I have taken back control of us and we are going to be ok because we are going to let Mother Nature's medicine re-shift and heal everything, every part of us that patriarchy manipulated and altered and changed. Even still, we will not have a natural menopause and it won't be easy, but at least we will have one! You in?!"

My body agreed with my soul and heart this was the right path for us and so the journey back to me, back to the woman I am, began. Again, it was a good thing I had no idea what to expect or I might have been too faint of heart to step onto this path. However, the warrioress within talked me through the night sweats and hot flashes, the loss of words right in the middle of teaching, the overall forgetfulness, the anger episodes and what I call the crazies. I learned though that my body was essentially having to grow a new way of being and not one that came equipped with the proper hormones, etc. for this time in a woman's life. I thank the Great

Mother Goddess, the Plant Spirits and my teachers and mentors for my learnings around Chickweed and Mugwort, Lemon Balm, Dandelion and Passionflower, Black Cohosh, Red Clover Vitex and more – my herbal allies that fed and nourished me for about 5 years. At that point, I was complete with some and others, especially Passionflower and Lemon Balm, still support me today. This choice to go 'au natural' was one of the hardest choices I ever made but absolutely one of the best!

Menopause is accepting being in the void. It is accepting being in the unknown and still being able to weave a vision of wholeness and completeness. It was my own Camino, and it took a lot of sitting with both the singularity and the all of nothingness and everything, separately and simultaneously.

Physically – especially for one surgically menopausal – it was relearning my body and what she wanted and needed.

Sometimes it was the most potent plant medicine I knew. Sometimes it was accepting that no matter how hard I tried – standing in front of a group of students – that the word or concept I wanted was NOT going to come! Sometimes it was an aphrodisiac and the healthiest food I could find. Many times, it was a whole carton of Haagen-Dazs Salted Caramel Ice Cream and/or Bailey's Irish Cream (sometimes both)! It was a reminder that everything had its own timing and purpose.

For me, menopause was many things beyond the limited idea of moving from the Mother directly to the Crone. Oh, I was asked at about 50 if I wanted a Croning ceremony and my answer was an emphatic NO! At that point, I hadn't even thought about going through my own menopause. Besides, what did I know at 50? I was asked again when I did enter Menopause, then at age 60 and again at age 65. Each time my reply was I don't feel ready to embody such wisdom and power.

Through this period, instead of being held to only three stages of a woman's life – one in which I never even participated – I found a plethora of new cycles and ways of being. I became the Phoenix and the Mystic, the Sorceress and Wild Witch Woman and many others before I reached Her…"Doesn't Give A Fuck Woman"… as my Soul opened to its own wild nature, perspective and way of being. This later stage now feels like where movement finally begins into the Hag, the Crone and then the Dark Mother and Death Mother.

Epilogue

Somewhere into the first year or so of teaching plant medicine and the beginnings of my natural menopause, I had a dream. I was working in a hospital that used only plant medicine and there was a woman who kept asking for me. When I finally went to her, she took my hand and said "I am so proud of you. You have done what I couldn't do, nor could my mother and I thank you." It was at that moment I realized this woman was MY mother and she was thanking me for reclaiming what surgical menopause had taken from three generations of women on the maternal side of my family – my grandmother, my mother and me. She was thanking me for calling out the horror of Patriarchy's theft of our natural female cycles AND in holy, sacred space ritualizing and reclaiming the beauty of how a woman's body and cycles are meant to be.

Arlene Bailey ©2022

Sacred Journey (Womb to Tomb)
Barbara O'Meara

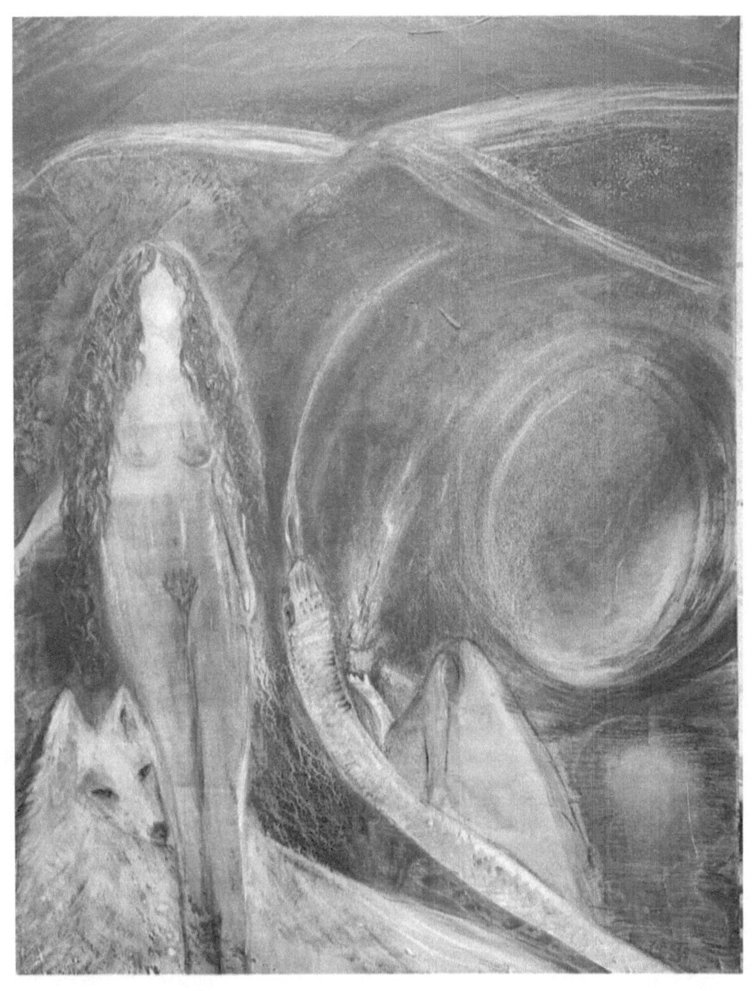

Holy Crone Crucible
Nuit Moore

They like to say we've
dried up, blossom withered,
fruit of vine waned to core.
They like to say we've
gone dry as bone,
as barren as desert,
hot heavy wind of void.
I'm here to tell you:
The desert doesn't belong to them.
They know not Her nature.
The gathered grandmothers
intuit the waning crescent,
dwell the terrain,
swell the oasis,
fill the vessels,
preserve the fruits,
tend the Tree of Life.
The nectar has gathered
towards the ripe interior-
for the truth is:
We are wells,
spinning holy
We are caves, descension deep
We are core, fierce mater lava.
Holy Crone Crucible.
Matrix magick.
We dwell and swell.
Reservoirs of revolution.
Sovereigns of intention.
Grandmothers of invention.

Life and Death
Liliana Kleiner

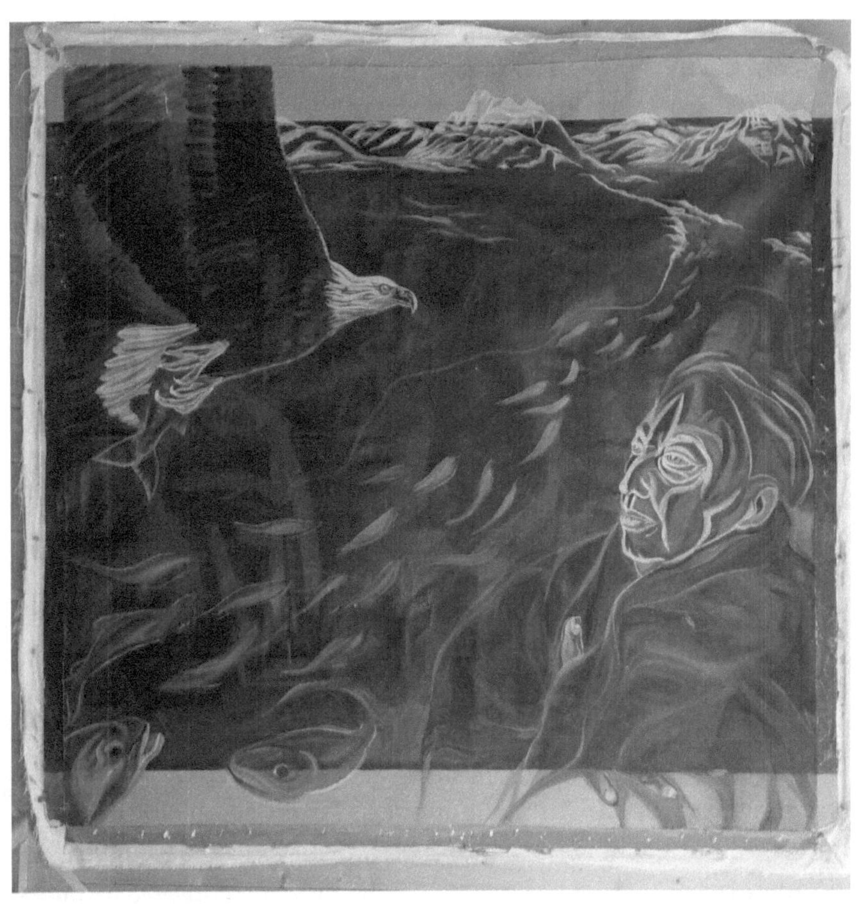

All Hail the Crone
Dr. Denise Renye

Cronehood, the third act of life, is a sacred time of a self-identified woman. Becoming a crone is not achieved merely by the passing of time and instead requires a rite of passage, an honoring of the new phase in a woman's life. When one is initiated into this phase, which follows maidenhood and motherhood, it's one of wisdom and unabashed confidence – the Crone no longer cares about judgment coming from others. Other people's opinions of her are really the business of those others. They are insignificant to her.

While she may notice an occasional waver within herself if judgment is slung at her, she has the wherewithal to pause, breathe, and find her connection point to Mother Earth. She is comfortable in herself, her identity, and who she is. She is in deep process allowing the conditioning that is inevitable in this lifetime to slough off as she moves through the trials and tribulations life has brought and brings her way. She is steady in her core. Dr. Jean Shinoda Bolen writes in *Crones Don't Whine:*

"Life gives you experience, and when you draw from it, that's true wisdom. By the time a woman is in her Crone years, she is in an amazing position to be an influence. To change things for the better, to bring what she knows into a situation, to be able to say, 'Enough is enough.' You don't have to just go along with things, which is often a part of the middle years [i.e., motherhood years]."

As a Crone, the woman is able to shine in all her glory and confidently crown herself in this third aspect of the Goddess: embodied maturity. Barbara Walker writes in her book *The Crone:*

"The Crone's title was related to the word crown and she represented the power of the ancient tribal matriarch who made the moral and legal decisions for her subjects and descendants. It was the medieval metamorphosis of the Wise Woman into the witch that changed the word Crone from a compliment to an insult and established the stereotype of malevolent old womanhood that continues to haunt elder women today."

In large part, the negative connotations associated with Crones come down to patriarchal trauma. Patriarchal trauma is the complex, multifold injury – psychological, social, emotional, spiritual, financial, and physical – associated with living under patriarchy, meaning the oppression and denigration of all things feminine that do not directly or indirectly cater to the traditional masculine. The traditional can sometimes be a mask for what is experienced as toxic. This toxicity embodies power over, callousness, and negative manipulation. Patriarchal trauma is any and all ways women, feminine expression and understanding, and the prioritization of relationality are told they're "less than," not allowed to be, or exist in this world even! Fear, judgment, belittling, covert and overt violence constitutes patriarchal trauma.

Covert violence can look like emotional abuse, which is yelling, putting a person down (belittling through discounting their words, ideas, and beliefs), commenting on their body, not respecting their boundaries (not hearing their "no"), and saying one thing while doing another. If someone requests space and time away from engaging in a conversation, or activity, and the other person will not hear the "no" but instead resorts to taunting, pushing harder, making fun of, or even humiliating, this is abuse. Saying "no" should be enough. No is a complete sentence, yet this has not been the learned experience of many women.

Abuse can also be verbal and along the lines of telling someone to "shut up" or nonverbal in terms of giving the silent treatment or pretending not to hear something accurately and making the other person repeat themselves numerous times.

And if a self-identified woman calls out this sort of behavior? An abuser might take the approach of gaslighting and either deny the behaviors outright or pin the blame on her. They might say, "You're too sensitive," or "You don't know what you're talking about. That didn't happen that way." The only reality that is "allowed" to exist is the abuser's version of reality. As we see, this happens to women all the time and with Crones, there is an extra kind of trauma that relates to her specifically.

Patriarchal trauma specifies that women are considered obsolete after a certain age (typically the few years preceding and entering into Cronehood) because they're no longer viewed as sexually desirable, as though they were mere objects for gazing upon and producing offspring for men and society at large. Traditionally, men do not contend with this issue. They are revered in roles in television and movies well into their elder years, seen as sages or silver foxes. Perhaps that's because biologically speaking, they are able to procreate throughout their life, not just during a specified time. But Crones? They're cast aside and if they're too vocal to be cast aside, they're considered bitches.

However, by reclaiming the power of the Crone, women in this stage of life can step into their wise-woman self. She is now a preserver of knowledge and bearer of wisdom acquired over a long life. We see this reflected in society with The Crone's Counsel, Raging Grannies, and Grandmothers for Peace International, groups where Crones are stepping into their role as social justice advocates and advisers. They have time and space to devote to causes that matter to them. Crones are healers and mentors.

In our youth-focused society, it can be difficult to claim the role of elder because by and large we're trying to preserve our youth. We live in a society wherein there is a high level of denial that aging is even a process we all undergo. With the normalization of plastic surgery and a wide array of other procedural options, we are able to engage in a shared delusion that youth is forever. It's something akin to a collective, widespread folie a deux, or a shared psychosis.

However, it wasn't always like that (and some societies like Native American tribes still value the role of elders). In ancient societies around the world, women were wisdom keepers, helping younger women bring new life into the world and helping older women as they exited this mortal realm. Marion Woodman reminds us in her book *Dancing in the Flames*, "The Crone has been missing from our culture for so long that many women, particularly young girls, know nothing of her tutelage. Young girls in our society are not initiated by older women into womanhood with its accompanying dignity and power. Without the Crone, the task of belonging to oneself, of being a whole person, is virtually impossible."

It used to be that the Crone enjoyed a special, revered status and was praised for her wisdom, healing skills, and moral leadership. That's because through the depths of her lived experiences she has a profound understanding of life and the world around her – she is a fount of wisdom for her community and a source of inspiration.
It's time to reclaim the power of the Crone while also recognizing the feelings that may arise when doing so. There may be grief about the life in the rear-view mirror. The grief may stem from victimizations, both acute and chronic, that have occurred throughout a long life. There are many subtle and not-so-subtle demeanings and aggressions that deserve to be grieved. It may be about the passing of friends, a partner, or the mere passage of time itself. Successful movement through grief is key in what makes a woman transition to Crone. A successful letting go, or surrendering, of what has passed so there is space created for rebirth of the new. There may be curiosity about what this new phase has in store for the Crone. There may be joy and celebration of what has been lived and what is yet to come. It's important to honor it all.

Each Crone differs in how she expresses herself, how she holds herself in this world. The Crone has the greatest opportunity – perhaps for the first time in her life – to embrace who she is. She can live the "not giving any more fucks about how she is perceived" life she has always dreamed of. With the fetters of this ever-present traumatized and traumatizing patriarchy, many may have to do this within and not make many changes without, but even acknowledging internally that she no longer cares about how she's perceived by others can begin to change the world. And taking a look around, it's obvious this world needs changing.

In my private practice as a psychologist and sexologist, I offer guidance through Cronehood ceremonies as part of my ritual and ceremonial psychology work. This is a fertile time and having a ritual carves out space for the sacredness that can be discovered. We start with a few preparation sessions, review what life has been like thus far and how the woman has gotten to where she is now, and then I facilitate the Crone ceremony itself, which can last anywhere from two to five hours. The ceremony includes altar creation, embodiment, song, acknowledgement of grief, and rebirth of the emboldened true self into Cronehood. This is followed up by a few integration sessions. These sessions help the woman go forward with her new, embodied sense of empowerment as the woman that she is.

Crones offer astounding and profound gifts to the world, purely by being themselves. If you are a Crone, I bow deeply to you and off you this gift. With outstretched hands, a meditation, and if you want to listen to the audio form, you may do so at www.wholepersonintegration.com/shoppe:

"I come to this part of my life as a Wise Woman who has been through so many trials, tribulations, successes, setbacks, and adventures. I am stronger now than I have ever been before. My body has been through so much and my mind has tackled so many problems and puzzles. And through it all, my spirit has exponentially gotten stronger. I am more connected with Source than ever and this shows up in my body as kundalini risings, which the mundane world calls hot flashes. The fires of the hot flashes allow space for me to access myself and Mother Earth all the way up the chakra channel through the center core of myself. My wild woman within can no longer be contained. She is not begging to be unleashed for she does not seek or require permission. She simply takes the space that is hers. I am she. She is me. I allow this process to unfold, trusting myself and the guidance I receive. I step into my role as mentor, embodying the sacred space just as I am. I. Am. Me. I am Crone."

References:

Shinoda Bolen, Dr. Jean. *Crones Don't Whine*. Berkeley: Conari Press, 2003.

Woodman, Marion. *Dancing in the Flames: The Dark Goddess in the Transformation of Consciousness*. Berkeley: Shambhala Publications, 1997.

Hecate Mask
Lauren Raine

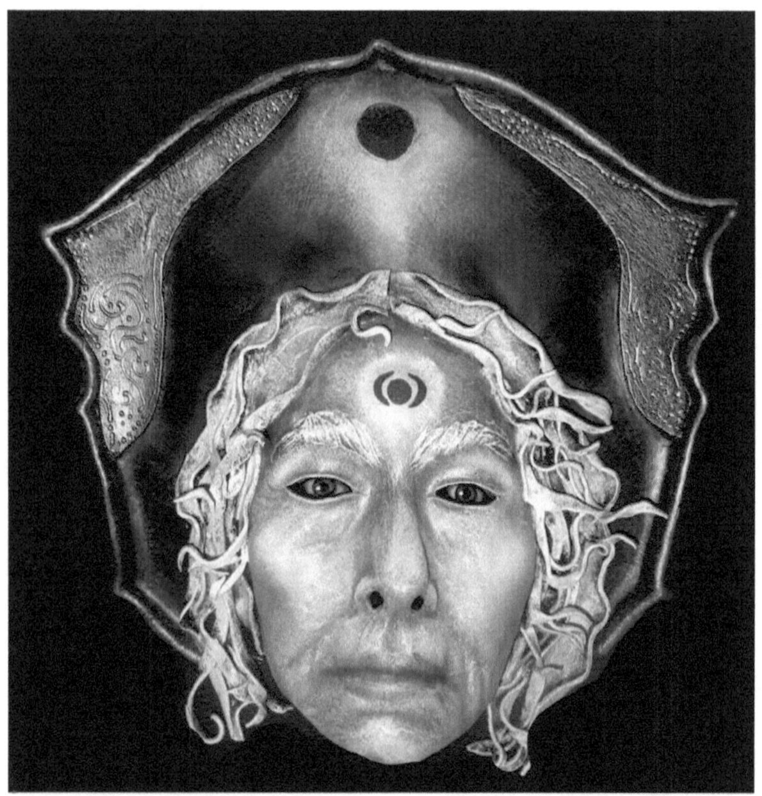

From The Masks of the Goddess Project.
masksofthegoddess.com

Hekate's Cool Moon
Janet Guastavino

In the arc of the heavens,
Hekate's cool moon hung
while winter ice sparkled
in the glimmer of its rays
and short shadows were cast by
ghosts and portents

In the crisp, cold air
Hekate stirred her cauldron
vapor rising from the brew
and brume ascending from the earth
—granddame and her daughter
bent to their respective tasks

In the chill of the season
Hekate glanced backwards,
beckoning us to follow
along the curved path
of well-trodden stones
to a place we had never seen

On that frost-tinged night,
Hekate's fading sliver of light
cast revelations on the landscape
And she, keeper of the knowing
that preceded mother and child,
was willing to share all with us

Midlife As Threshold, Initiation and Rite of Passage
Laura Valenti

I would like to acknowledge the place from which I am speaking: I am a white, straight, able-bodied and privileged woman in Europe. As such, what I offer here is based on my experience and will not be relevant or resonant for all women everywhere. BIPOC women, lesbian and transgender women, women living in differently-abled bodies, women with different cultural backgrounds will have a different experience from mine and I do not mean to suggest that what follows is exhaustive on the topic or a one size fits all. I am aware of the challenges to include complex topics such as patriarchy and the need to recognise it as an internalised system of oppression to which we also contribute. Nevertheless, I invite you to take this journey with me.

In our contemporary Western society, many people think that midlife and the time between perimenopause and menopause (and all that comes with it) is a curse. Furthermore, this time of life is highly pathologised. As women, we also tend to believe that we lose our most important job or function: to give life. We become useless. Powerless. Hopeless. The best time of life is gone.

Our culture normalises and promotes disconnection from our bodies and souls. It offers us chemical pills and quick fixes instead. As a response to such distortion, we may end up feeling even more doomed, confused, lost, and exiled from ourselves. We may think that we're destined to lose youth, vitality, and beauty, and as such, our life will never be the same. It's all we can do to just get by.

If, like me, you've experienced many ups and downs in this journey, sometimes you may feel that you are going mad or there is a fracture in your psyche. We blame ourselves, our unresolved traumas, core wounds, limiting beliefs, hormones and think that we have not done enough therapy, healing work and ultimately failed spectacularly at taking care of ourselves or manifesting the life we want. This process can be debilitating and isolating. But if we choose to, it can become a journey into the most hidden and buried corners of our being and a true adventure.

For some of us, this voyage becomes an exploration of the dark night of the soul.

We may face physical, mental, emotional, and spiritual turmoil, while we are also bombarded by media, dogmas, polarised views, and medical mainstream ideas or laws that undermine our bodily autonomy and right to decide (the anti-abortion legislation in Texas is just a recent example). From photo-shopped images of skinny bodies with big boobs to Barbie faces, glamorous selfies on social media, inauthentic stories of success, TV advertisements of beauty products, plastic surgery, and expensive fashion items, we are constantly reminded of the endemic fear of death in our consumerist society and the myth of the eternal youth. As you know, the list does not end here. Something insidious is planted in our consciousness.

The message is clear. There is something wrong with us.

We are not enough. We lack something. We need to do more. Our body is imperfect and objectified. We need more possessions. That cream, pill, guru, or shoes will fix us or fill the void inside us.

We face the impossible task of meeting the cultural standards that dictate how we need to look, behave, feel, and appear. Women are familiar with this kind of pressure. Too fat, too skinny, too successful, too anonymous, too bold, too shy, too extroverted, too introverted, too busy, too relaxed.

To an extent, historically, it was a curse to be born in a female body and have a menstrual cycle. How many of us hold a positive memory of our first menarche? How many associations are there between blood, shame and disgust? Since childhood, we may have interiorised that feeling that there is something terribly wrong, faulty or even dirty at our core. We must be inherently bad.

The picture becomes even more distorted if we think about sexuality.

I grew up in a traditional Italian Catholic context. I remember from a young age rebelling intuitively against the two main archetypes related to women: the saint and the whore. Alongside that, the most powerful culturally interiorised and accepted was the martyr. There was something noble and sublimated about sacrificing one's happiness, needs, joy, intuition, power, and overall health.

Furthermore, I remember when I came across Pliny's work in my late twenties and discovered what he wrote about menstrual blood:

"Contact with [menstrual blood] turns new wine sour, crops touched by it become barren, grafts die, seed in gardens are dried up, the fruit of trees fall off, the edge of steel and the gleam of ivory are dulled, hives of bees die, even bronze and iron are at once seized by rust, and a horrible smell fills the air; to taste it drives dogs mad and infects their bites with an incurable poison."

I feel enraged if I sense how much self-loathing, shame and self-hatred has been passed from one generation onto the other based on these assumptions and beliefs about women's bodies.

We carry behind us at least two thousand years of linear thinking and history written by patriarchy and systems of oppression. Luckily, women have been always gathering, often in secret, to keep our art, craft, poetry, wisdom, magic, medicine, songs, dances and intuition alive.

And whether we've had the opportunity to explicitly meet like this in our lifetime, we do carry these gifts of memory, visions and knowledge in our bones, psyche, dreams, and genes.

There is always an opportunity to meet women who want to travel alongside you and share a deep heart and soul connection.

We may ask what is at stake here? What is going to happen if this pivotal time of midlife is going to simply be labelled as something awful, uncomfortable, to be ashamed of and nothing more?

I think if that were to be the case, we would go in a dangerous direction, where we could lose part of our humanity and essence that are utterly needed in this historical moment. I think the life of our soul is at stake here. Our role as wisdom keepers and life protectors are at stake. Our future on the planet is at stake. Our relationship with our younger girls is at stake. Ultimately, our physical, mental, emotional, and spiritual health is at stake. Our ancestral wisdom could be lost. Ancient songs, stories and whispers could be forgotten.

The more we disconnect from our bodies as a sacred temple, the more we disconnect from the living earth and Her rhythms, living wisdom and cycles.

Intuitively, despite the messages that tell us otherwise, we know that (especially at the threshold of midlife) we need to follow our intuition, inner compass, wisdom, dreams, and visions. We need to land in our bodies softly while we also get to know ourselves at the most deeply intimate and cellular level. Midlife is a fluid time, where we move with our waters, ups and downs, inward and outward, into the depths of our oceanic being, slowly and fiercely.

We learn to embrace stillness whilst learning to flow with ease. We swim with paradoxes. We become the calm lake and the thunder. We are the drop of rain and the ocean. We may experience utter despair and the most exquisite beauty at the same time, knowing that we are constantly transforming ourselves. We dance with polarities.

This is a time when we sit in the alchemical fire of initiation. We can play with metaphors and images to create a new and uplifting narrative around midlife. If we imagine that when the flames meet the water, we enter a highly chaotic and somewhat destructive time, we can tap into ancient archetypal forces and a circular sense of time. It is like being with the power of a volcano, powerful steam, lava, or the Goddess Kali. The encounter between water and fire is the most creative and transformative.

Midlife is also time for rest, guidance, synchronicities, and dissolving taboos. Some call it a sacred pause. Others refer to it as a second Spring. Some women may prefer to see it as Autumn. I like to think of it also as a radical time, because this word comes from *radicalis,* in Latin which means 'originating in the ground or root'. In the seventeen century the figurative meaning was 'going to the origin, essential'. I see in this cycle of life the possibility to fully land into our bodies and reclaim our essence. Sometimes I imagine myself growing into and from the ground as a plant.

Some other women emphasise the rebirth process that takes place. The old makes space for the new. The phoenix rises.

And yet, we must remember that rebirth follows death. So this is also a time for dying. Shedding skin. Dissolution. Because to an extent, we enter into more contact at the visceral level with our mortality. We are going to die. We are going to lose loved ones. That is the only certainty in the great sea of the unknown. And this can be extremely disorienting for our psyche because in our industrialised countries we have removed our relationship with natural life cycles, including death. We've lost our collective rituals and severed our connection from the web of life in which we are embedded and upon which our life depends.

Midlife is a time where we encounter the great void. The unknown. The Mystery. The lack of control. The fragility of life and its sheer beauty and preciousness. The ego screaming and wanting to be in charge. The prayers to let go and surrender. The losses. The grief. The rage. The broken dreams. Health challenges.

I feel that this journey into midlife is a prayer.

Sometimes, when we are exhausted (after trying all sorts of healing and therapeutic modalities) and we have done all we could to feel better, all that is left is to open up our psyche and soul to the possibility of deep surrender. Just to feel and be. No need to perform or achieve anything. So, our bones can rest too. Maybe it is about whispering to our soul 'you can let go, you can relax' so our body can hear that too and can soften a bit more.

Maybe this is about resting on the ground and doing nothing. Maybe it's about listening to the whispers of the wind, answering to the songs of the birds, and letting our weight sink into the ground. Maybe it's about being in silence. Maybe it's about letting our inner child know that she is held, safe, accepted, welcome, protected. Perhaps the cicadas are singing for you too today, saying 'you are loved my child, you are a child of the Earth'.

Maybe it's about trusting the synchronicities and not dismissing the flight of an eagle hovering upon our head, the branches of the trees moving when we feel in telepathic loving conversation with them, or the appearance of the tiniest insect on our doorstep. Perhaps we can remember that it is only in recent history that the Earth is seen as an inanimate object when in reality, she can hear us and is in constant communication and relationship with us if we are willing to listen.

I think that we need to reclaim midlife as a sacred time of reflection, healing, community making and introspection.

Many of us may question our identities, jobs, relationships, old patterns and limiting beliefs. There is something powerful about accepting that we need to let go of that which is not serving us anymore and learn more about surrendering. And I also think that we need to do this together, with other women. It does not need to be a lonely and isolating path.

From children leaving home to not having children, changing home or not having a home, divorce, losses, wanting more purpose, meaning, love and connection, many of us fall on our knees while we come back home to ourselves, listening to what truly matters and our hearts. Those places of not knowing, grief, sometimes rage, exhaustion (especially for those of us who've been working with our inner world for many years) are all portals into surrender. Nothing else can be done. There is nothing more to lose. It is a place where we choose whether we want to trust life at the most intimate level and face our deepest fears.

It is not an easy task to reframe stories about midlife. Especially when there are also physiological changes occurring in the body, from hormonal adjustments to sleeping patterns, mood swings, hot flashes, weight gain. You name it. Often, we are not educated about how to navigate these challenges in a way that is empowering, uplifting, and dignifying.

To tell a story about midlife as a threshold, initiation and rite of passage means that you and I can rise in dignity. We can find comfort where previously there was despair, power in the places of powerlessness, beauty, and poetry in the ugliness and ultimately, we can celebrate our rebirth and precious life. We are not meant to do it alone, but in circles, with sisters and elders, with songs, prayer, and dances. We can lift each other up. This is a magical time to dream awake our future and envision who we want to be. We can welcome and embody our wildest, wisest, and radical self joyfully, softly, outrageously and with grace.

You Were Meant to Bloom
Caroline Selles

I am a bouquet of paper flowers
A dry forest, whose flowers want to bloom, but have forgotten how
Dry flowers
That crumble when touched
like fake beauty
Dusty, dry flowers in a neglected waiting room,
Not fresh and
Growing wild in a lush tropical isle

My healing must begin with these flowers
The flower of my feminine self
This must be the focus
All else is window coverings,
Changing the drapes and moving the furniture
While the foundation cracks,
And the roof leaks

All else, is a band-aid on a broken, bruised soul
My healing begins when I stop blaming myself,
For what happened

A rose wants to bloom
Wild and free
It does not want to be
Picked, dead and dried.

Sacred Wisdom
Liliana Kleiner

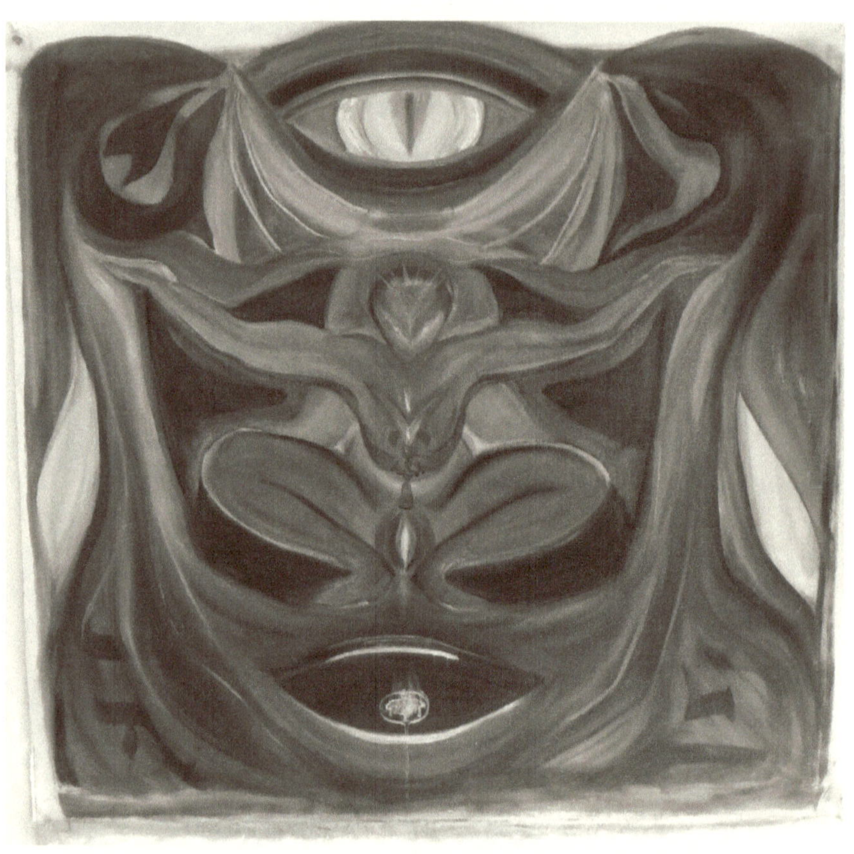

The Deeper Meaning of Blood
Rhonda Melanson

I've crawled
through this hazy district
blood memories on my back.

I've been pricked
buckets poured over my head
buried and found again
an afterbirth
pressed grapes
aged wine.

Look how tomato sun
clots my wounds
into perfect body art
jewels for a kingdom
without pain.

I no longer fear red.

Crone Goddess
Caroline Selles

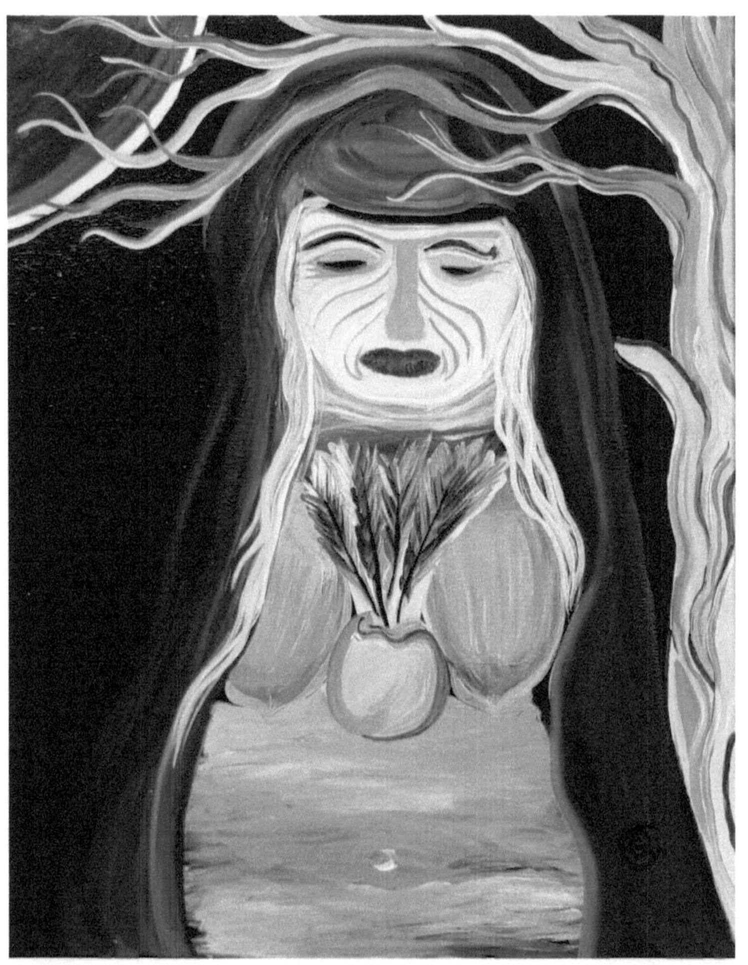

When I was still in grade school, just at the cusp of puberty, I was violently and sexually traumatized by a licensed medical professional. Immediately afterward, this MD told me I likely had Polycystic Ovarian Syndrome and would "never have children". I do believe the words, combined with the severe physical trauma became manifested as my destiny. I suffered with horrible hormonal disorders and sexual dysfunction and shame for years and ultimately experienced early menopause in what should have been the prime of my mothering years. When I began to heal with Goddess, I had to come to terms with this loss, the violence and the infertility. I went from Maiden to Crone, without ever experiencing the Mother.

My words and my art are my children. They stand as testament to my creative power. These three poems reflect the evolution of my coming to terms with my past as I embrace my future and the gifts of the Crone Goddess. I no longer feel that my sense of femininity or sexuality must end, just because my cycles did. In many ways, they are just beginning.

Perimenopausal
Caroline Selles

A dying rose.
I've never even bloomed, and I'm
Already withering.
Never a mother,
I have not owned my feminine power.
Yet,
I am about to lose it.

Goddess energy.
I need Goddess energy.

Silent Night
Caroline Selles

I could do without the cold
But the silence, well
There is something there
Shadows come out to play
Muses dance just beyond the flickering candle flame
Internal electricity sparks
A smile begins to curl upon my lips
My eyes would shine brightly if you could see them
Old women and ancient spirits love the night
The silent night
A night full of magic and promises yet to come
Listen dear one
Be not distracted by the light
For the silent night holds all the dreams, secrets and
Pleasures you long to know
Revel in the silence
Dance with the shadows
Listen to the whisperings
They will make you a dream
A dream that floods your soul
And fills the silent night with laughter

The Caillech Mask
Lauren Raine

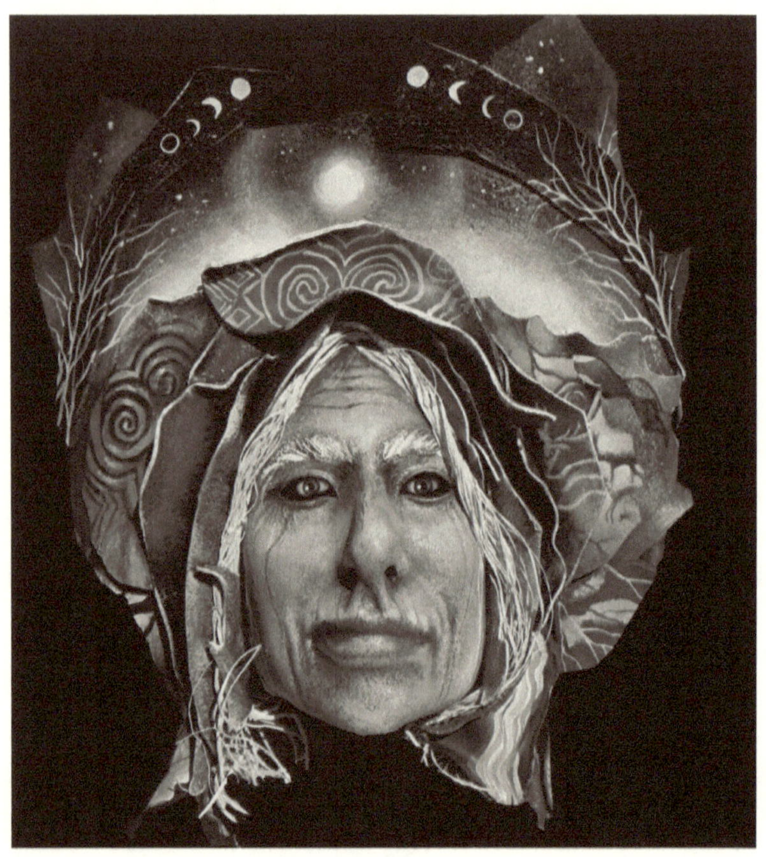

From The Masks of the Goddess Project.
masksofthegoddess.com

Gifts from an Cailleach
Ger Moane

In the Irish tradition, an Cailleach, the Crone Goddess, is as old as the hills. She is Earth Goddess, originator of life who dwells in every grain of soil, in the roots and leaves, plants and trees.

Animals – cow, deer, wolf – are her companions. She is the giant who creates and shapes the landscape with her huge hands that can carry boulders and powerful legs that can leap from hilltop to hilltop. Long-lived, she has been here from the beginning of time, through epochs of earth-time and lifetimes of humans. She is wild and magical, a shapeshifter who can appear as a wizened old woman or as a bright young woman. In Irish Celtic myth, she is the Goddess who tests and confers sovereignty on the earthly king. In legend and folklore, she most often appears as a hag, often with grey hair and long fingernails, free to live alone in the mountains, to impart a lesson or a warning, for she is fierce and protective of her charges.

All over Ireland there are standing stones and cairns called after her, said to have been created by her as she moved over the landscape with an apron full of stones. One of the most magical places still bears her name in the Irish language – Sliabh na Cailliagh, which translates as the Hill of the Cailleach (also called Loughcrew in English). There are two high hills at Sliabh na Cailliagh, each with a cairn on top which from a distance look like two breasts. Each cairn is a mound of earth and stone about 30 feet high which covers a passageway leading into an inner chamber where there is beautiful Neolithic art carved on the stones – spirals, circles and other symbols of Earth Goddess and the cycle of life. Outside is a huge stone seat called 'The Hag's Chair', associated in folklore and tradition with augury and inspiration from an Cailleach.

It was here that I had my crone initiation. I was called to attend a weekend of women gathering to honor Cronehood and an Cailleach with the guidance of Irish druid Annette Beard and bean feasa (Wise Woman) Cait Brannigan. Whether I was called or sent is unclear to me. I had pushed through menopause, reframing hot flushes as power surges, but I was also flustered, disconnected, and sometimes depressed and incapable. I didn't really connect with Crone energy until I was diagnosed with breast cancer a few years into menopause. That was really a shock. I felt as if my body had betrayed me, and my trust and confidence in everything, including Goddess energy, was shattered. Menopause and getting older felt like a threat where anything might happen and illness might stalk me, where I was no longer sure of who I was and where my life was going. Fortunately, I had been practicing Irish shamanism for several years and just at my lowest ebb, after the diagnosis, I received a wonderful gift of land from the universe that seemed like happenstance but of course was more. I knew was from Her. At the time I didn't have a name for her as the Crone Goddess, an Cailleach. But she was calling me, asking me to take the time to open to her, and to the other Goddesses of Irish Celtic Mythology.

And so, I gathered with the other women for an afternoon at the cairn on the hilltop dedicated to an Cailleach. We stood in half circle with a breeze blowing by the entrance to the cairn. Annette and Cait called in the elements and the four directions along with animal and spirit guides. Those of us who were moved to do so stepped forward to enter the cairn. We stood at the threshold and awaited permission to enter. Soon a group was gathered in the inner chamber. Soft candlelight illuminated the carvings on the stones. We journeyed together to drumming. Suddenly, out of the darkness, an Cailleach appeared to me – she told me she was the mother of our people, and her bright light filled me with joy and hope. In that moment of illumination, my fears about my changing body, about my health and about my future faded. My trust restored, I felt inspired by the strength and power of her aged yet ageless body.

Over the years since I have visited Sliabh na Cailliagh many times, and felt her presence through journeying, meditation and writing about ancient spirituality in the form of a novel. She has walked with me through treatment, recovery, and prolonged menopause, moving me to set aside the patriarchal denigration of older women and follow a path of connection to ancient wisdom, where the bodily changes that come with menopause, serious illness and aging offer new possibilities for ways of being. Irish Goddesses can be elusive, presenting as fluid energy weaving through stories rather than as a fixed personage. The stories about them in mythology, like in other mythologies, often strip them of agency and involve dismemberment and sexual violence. I have only come to feel and know an Cailleach (and Brigid, Boann, Macha, Morrigan, Eriu, and other Irish Goddesses) through dreaming, journeying to their sacred sites, celebrating in ritual, sitting with their stories and opening to their energies. Cailleach teaches that the passage of time is not a lessening but a transformation, a letting go that opens space for deeper connection to our soul's purpose.

Spark us, oh Cailleach, oh wild one,
let our bodies and souls be open to you
Let us carry the torch, keep your light alive
Let us animate the changes we need so that your power may rise
Buíochas – thank you.

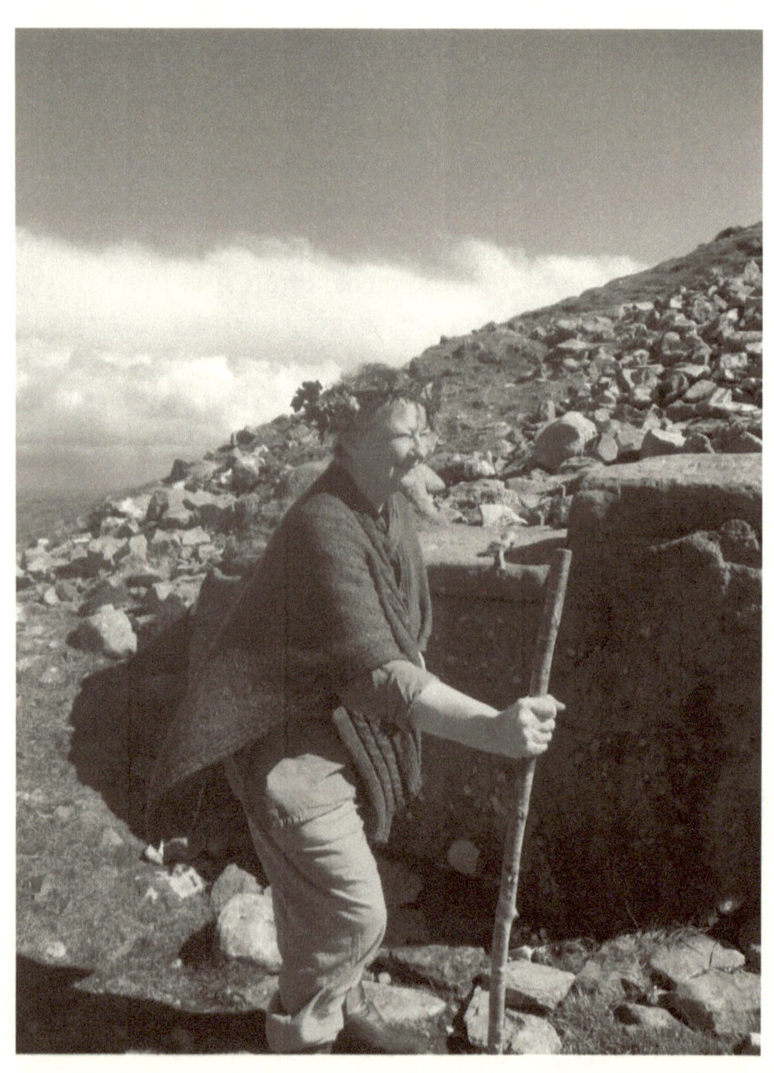

Reclaiming the Holy Hag
Nuit Moore

"You're a f*cking hag!" he spit at me with hate.

I was 25 years old, a radiant bloom. He was my boyfriend at the time, and of course he called me all the other things that abusers call women: bitch, cunt, whore (and no, he didn't last long – I sent him to jail a few days later when it turned physical, and it was done). All those words intended to batter my insides. But his verbal arrows of woman-hate deflected off me as weak and powerless over me as he was.

For you see, I was a feminist – and not only a feminist – but a FEMINIST WITCH.

And I knew the original roots of these words, and I knew their original power.

And I have reclaimed those words and that power every single time those arrows have been shot my way – as slice-sharp as some of them wanted to be.

But I confess – being called a hag at 25 was so utterly unexpected, that I considered it with a relish after the surprise of it. Because Hag is a particularly potent word in relation to female power and female wisdom, and especially elder female power and wisdom. It has also been used historically to invalidate and uglify that female power and wisdom in women of and over a certain age. At 25, I found it rather hilarious at the core of it to be called Hag, and I claimed it with glee.

I'm 50 now – twice the age of when I first experienced being called a Hag. And I've meditated on how that would feel, at 50, to have that arrow come at me now. Would it sting a little now that I edge the cusp of coming Cronehood? Now that I am no longer that fresh radiant bloom that could laugh in the face of it? Would it pierce me finally now, that arrow of misogyny?

It sure as Hel would not! I would still receive it with glee, and on top of that, I would hail Her!

Yes, I hail the Holy Hag!

The Holy Hag is a portal of POWER. A power that terrifies the Patriarchy, and has for centuries upon centuries. The Holy Hag is so powerful that those men who oversaw the witch hunts of Europe and early America, in the crucible of their murderous misogyny, were hellbent on turning the Hag into an epithet of female evil.

As a result, the word Hag has long translated to an 'ugly evil old woman', a meaning heavy with that brutal misogyny. But Hag as a word has roots in two ancient Saxon forms: the words haegtessa (Middle English) and hagzussa (Old High German), both which mean witch and hedge-rider (a shamanistic practitioner associated with the Cunning Craft/witchcraft). The words Hexe and Haxe are also related, both meaning 'witch/witchcraft'. The practices associated with the origins were oracular and shamanistic in nature.

These words only later carried a specific mantle of malevolence as the result of that merciless misogyny that drove the horrifying witch hunts of the 14th-17th centuries. The Witch Craze of this time period heavily focused on accusing women of devil worship and witchcraft, and in particular danger were older women, who were usually portrayed as twisted, malevolent agents of the Dark Arts. The historian Lyndal Roper states "The witch-hunt had offered a clear way of dealing with evil by locating the source of evil within an old woman.

Old women were disproportionally represented among the victims of the witch craze; and the old woman was the abiding stereotypical witch."[17] Although the witch-craze was (in most part) over by the 1800's, to this day the popular mainstream representation of a Witch is an old, ugly woman, bent on maleficence – or, as it is still widely connotated, a "hag."

Another etymological source I like to consider is the Ancient Greek word *hagios*, which means 'Holy, to be venerated' – as expressed in the Hagia Sophia, which means 'Holy Wisdom' (and is what I always invoke before doing a reading with my cards). The Gnostic Sophia is the feminine face of God, and Sophia as a Goddess /archetype in feminist spirituality has come to represent the wisdom of women, and older women especially. Thus, Hagia Sophia is literally Holy Female Wisdom. Although there is no proven link that I know of between the word Hag with Hagia, I cannot help but personally consider it a possible connection.

The reclaiming of the original roots and meanings of the words that have been twisted to invalidate female power is an act of magick, and a potent activism. In my experience, doing so shines the shield, turns the mirror, burns the bindings. In the reclaiming of the Holy Hag, I have personally been set on a path of liberation rather than lament as I arc towards the cusp of Cronehood.

It is a powerful blessing to have this awareness of the truth of the Holy Hag, both in an internal and external way. The truth of the roots of female power, red with the life-giving blood of women.

Remembering too the roots red with the blood of the harrowing number women killed in the name of brutal, relentless misogyny. The legacy of the Hag is powerful beyond belief, and we must both remember and reclaim it. To reclaim the Holy Hag, to hail Her and to honor Her is indeed an act of deep and true magick, and a

---

[17] Roper, Lyndal. *The Witch in the Western Imagination.* Studies in Early Modern German History. Charlottesville VA: University of Virginia Press, 2012.

particularly potent activism.

As for me, I hail Her in every incoming new strand of glittery hair, in every new crease of skin like a journey on a map. I hail Her in my empty nesting widowhood solitude, the gifts of which are as delicious as honey, often overriding the little bitter bits. I hail Her in the softness of my belly and the gravity of my breasts. I hail Her with every Dark Moon held deep within my womb. I hail Her coming into view in my mirror, even as I walk my journey currently as Empress. I hail Her in my set boundaries, which my inner Hag fiercely defends. I hail Her in the name of all my elder ancestors, of all my Grandmothers. And I hail Her in honoring my own hard earned Wise Woman wisdom, like a cauldron richly seasoned with every passing year.

Thinking on all this has me looking back on my journey to this cusp of Cronehood. Thinking of the debts of gratitude that I have towards the Crones and Hags that have inspired me continuously over the last three decades. These fierce and beautiful firebrands that have fostered in me this anticipating excitement of my own incoming time as Crone. In a society where women are still constantly assaulted with negative reinforcement in becoming an older and elder woman – in becoming a "hag" – to have this invaluable vision of the older and elder woman as the vibrant powerhouse of wisdom and magick that she is, is a treasure beyond measure. It is my hopes that one day, this will be the norm rather than the exception. We must continue collectively to work our acts of magick, our acts of potent activism.

So let us Hail the Holy Hag together! Hail! Hail the Holy Hag!

Reclaiming the Holy Hag
Nuit Moore

*#3 in a series reclaiming
the Holy Hag.*

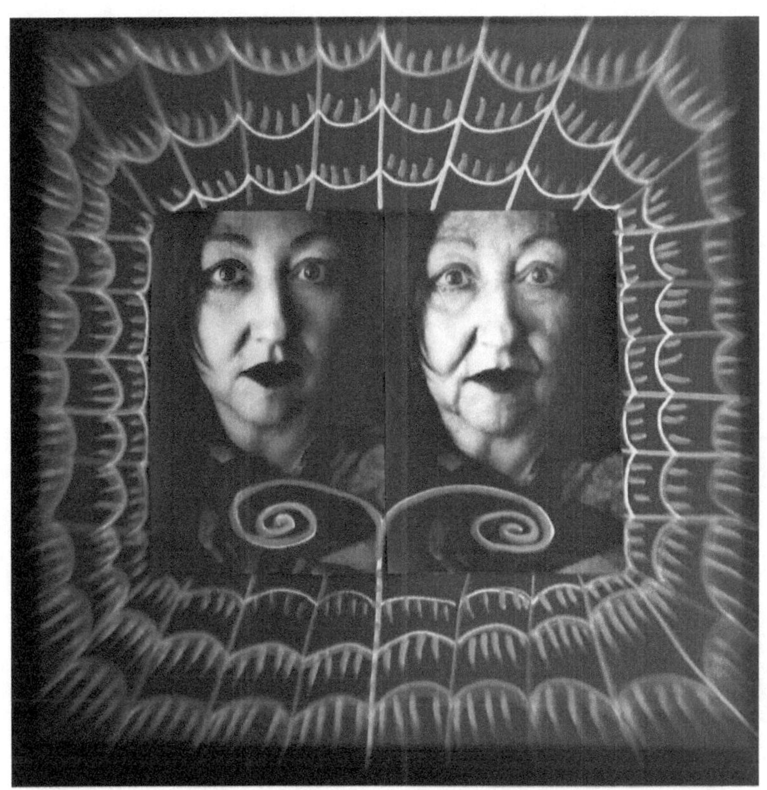

*A self-portrait – one recent,
the other future (via age progression).
My scarlet cord,
my wombic web,
metaformic.*

Caw of a Crow
Hayley Arrington

Any crone worth her salt Is accompanied by a crow.
One or two for good measure.

Crows' raucous caws Garner attention
Like unwanted company.

Crones, like caws,
Are also unwanted.
They interrupt the flow—

Even if just in the backyard
And not in a forest, dark,
Where Crones met
and caws heard
instill a bone-deep fear.

Any backyard-dwelling crone
Will tell you that she,
Too, instills this fear.

Her lines of living Say, "You will die"
More loudly than a crow's caw.

But no one listens to her
Or to the caws that say,
"I'll eat your tongue when I find you dead."

Portal-Power-Perimenopause
Nuit Moore

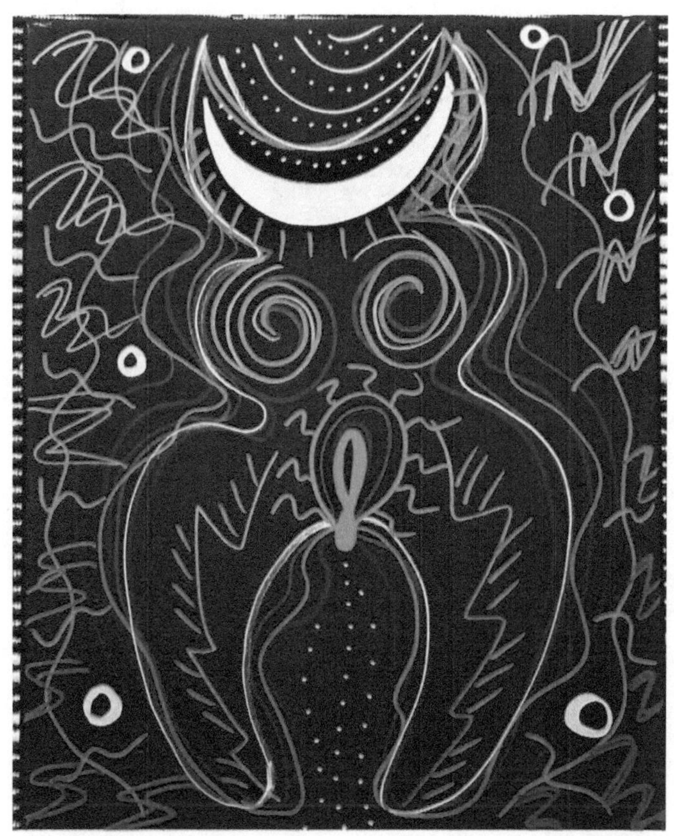

*'Portal-Power-Perimenopause' is a trance painting done in 2021
during a phase of particularly fiery hot flashes. Here is my abstract
form activated on high in what I have affectionately named
'Kuntalini Rising'; yonic and wombic power vitalized at the
root core within the alchemical process of perimenopause.*

Not Yet a Crone
Hayley Arrington

I am not yet a Crone
but I aspire to be.
I am middle-aged,
caught between longing for youth
and fearing death,
yet glad I've neither.

In the mirror,
I see her waiting,
a hint of women older,
some gone to their final rest,
and I hope to meet her someday,
she who smiles and waits.

I am not yet a Crone
but I aspire to be.
I let my crone
weave silver threads through my hair
and paint dancing crow's feet around my eyes
as she waits the passing seasons
for her own time.

Explosive Birthing
Kay Louise Aldred

I was not quiet when I gave birth. I cursed, shouted, groaned, and bellowed. I swore. I was primal, untamed, and uninhibited. My VOICE opened in tandem with my womb. SHE WAS HEARD. No one could argue. Everyone looked a little bit afraid.

The power of my body was beyond my control. I felt inhabited, by a force, an energy current, a fire flow, which was unstoppable, relentless, and unharnessed. I ripped off my clothes; I was animalistic and predatory.

Childbearing in a state of trauma and dissociation – mentored and prepared for the experience in an 'intellectual' way by mainstream medicine – resulted in the three childbirths causing further trauma and somatic desensitisation in an area of my body already impacted by sexual abuse.

I wish I had understood my body and the primordial Feminine like I do now, then. I wish maternity services were trauma informed and trained.

What is happening for me in Perimenopause is a reclamation of birthing. Healing the womb and vulva is part of this, sensitising tissues and going 'back', somatically to labour; the contractions, the crowning, the push, to reconnect to the fire flow and POWER of explosive birthing – safely.

This is happening organically. I did not consciously decide to do it. It is unfolding as I birth creatively and become more internally Self leading and am seen and heard as my authentic self.

Womb of the Earth
Katrina Stadler

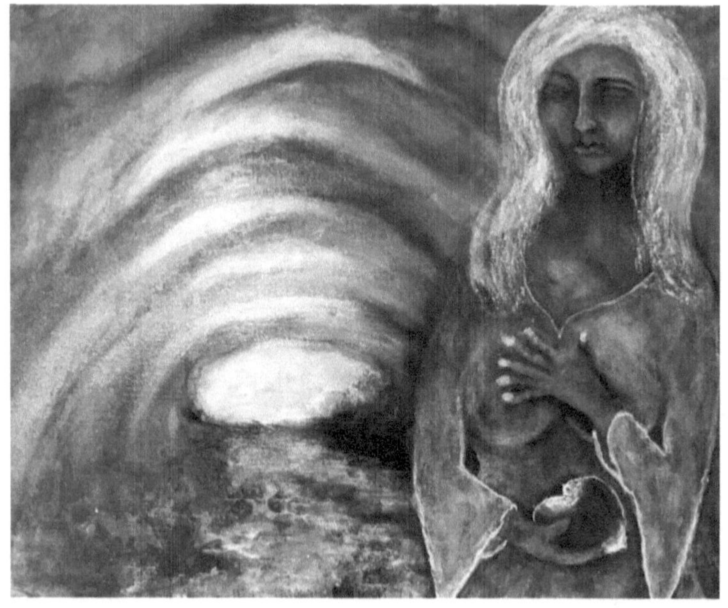

She Has Come
to Redraw the Circle
Kaia Maeve Tingley

She has come to redraw the circle.
She has come in our time of need.
She has come renewing connections.
She has come to plant the seeds.
She has come to bathe us in rhythm.
She has come, depraved and divine.
She has come to heal the schism.
She has come to change our minds.

Death is a lady we could learn to revere.
She might seem far off until She comes near.
One day She will find you, whisper in your ear.
Her lesson for you? Don't waste your time here.
There is no such thing as an enemy or friend.
There is no such thing as a beginning or end.
There is no such thing as being alone,
we all come from Mama Earth, and to Her, we'll go home.

She did not come to serve your purpose.
She did not come to fill your gaze.
She did not come to make you happy.
And she's not going to listen when you say, behave!
Give thanks for the days you get to exist.
Be love. Be passion. Be sacred bliss.
Plug-in let your roots go down deep to below
Surrender, allow, become part of the flow.

Yeah, she has come to tear the house down,
The giant house of make-believe,
That needy people have built upon Her,
Despite millions of warnings that we've all received.

She has come with sacred rage,
To burn the false gods that now sit on the stage.

She has come to school the children,
With a wise old book from a much older age.

She has come to teach us respect.
To surrender the things we have come to expect.
She has come to pass on Her knowledge.
She has come to shuffle the deck.
She has come; She doesn't care if you want Her.
She has come because Her time is here.

She has come because SHE wants to.
The great circle both ends and begins right here.
She has come to reclaim the night.
She has come to feed the soil.
She has come to dismantle your armor.
She has come to let you feel.
She has come to break old systems.
She has come to stroke your fear.
She has come to heal the wounds.
She has come. The Goddess is here.

Morrigan
Andrea Redmond

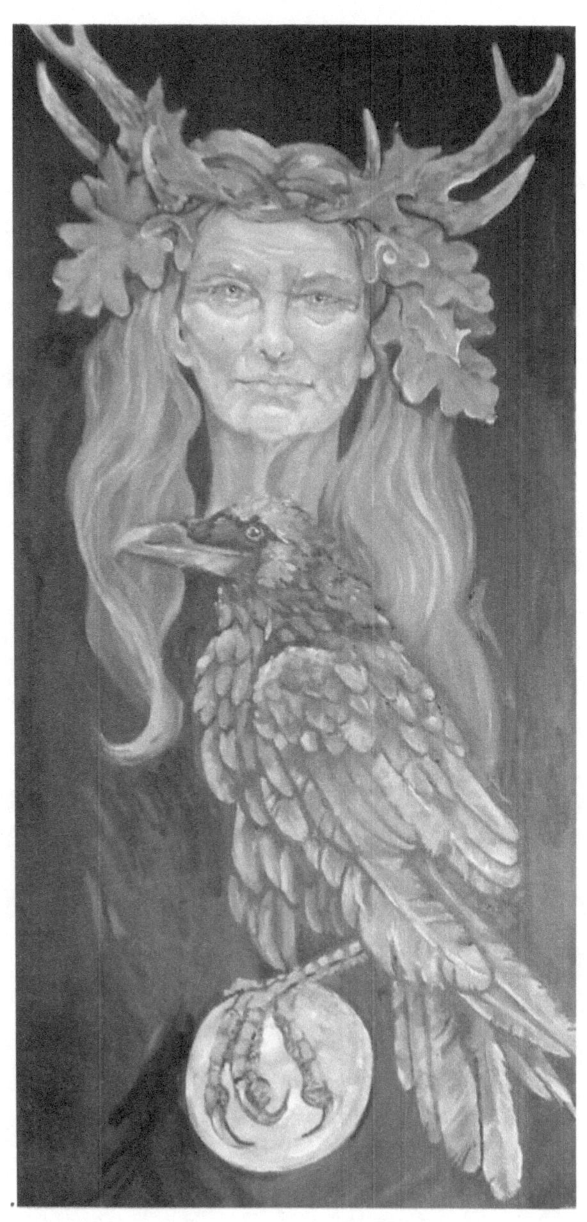

Autumn
Mary Lane

Autumn is when there is a slow build-up to an orgasmic eruption of a brilliantly colored display of celebration of a life cycle well honoured.

It is when life and death come together with an embrace of oneness, a recognition of love and service to the whole as the trees let go of leaves they nourished. The plants drop their seeds into a well-prepared bed for their gestation into a new life cycle.

It is when Mother earth says, it's time to move towards a much-needed rest. I have done well in providing, nourishing, and holding this incarnation of life. Now, it's time for me.

But, as I rest, as I let go, as I die back, even in death, I feed life.

As a crone in the autumn of my life, who is also an expression of nature, the Mother, I ponder, reflect, inquire, what is my human expression of all this? What does my autumn look and feel like? How can I align with the larger expression?

How can I celebrate and honor my life cycle? How can I let go with the grace of the trees? How can my death support life?

How can I walk in an ecstatic embrace of life and death, holding one another, together, in celebration of both, knowing there is no either or, no longer divided. Together, in never ending cycles of love. How can I be fully alive, embracing it all, before my body's death?

As a crone, in the autumn of my life, I have outgrown the childish antics of patriarchal lies, to get its way. I can no longer be fooled by a story that dismisses what I can see, experience, and feel before my very eyes and heart, as the life and death cycles unfold around and within me. I am here, expressing and celebrating the wisdom garnered from a well lived life cycle on this never-ending journey, that is now in the autumn season of another incarnation.

Well, I have better things to do than vie for your approval of an elderly woman, according to your made-up story. This foolishness about our need to fear death I intend to dispel the spell.

I have lived through many life and death cycles in this incarnation and know the folly of such lies. I stand before you, and take my well-earned seat, not at your table, but at the table of our Great Mother, so I too can feed life with my death.

I'm in the autumn of my life, officially a crone. I sit at the table where I am honored and celebrated, orgasmically embracing all the flavors of life and death, deep within my own soul, preparing to imbue our world with a natural expression of love inherent in my very nature, my final gift of this incarnation, as my death feeds life, with the energy that will birth a world we have all longed to embody once again. Yes, you were wise to fear me. For I have freed myself from childish patriarchal antics. I have even reclaimed my death. And I can transform the world by just being me, the crone.... Mother Nature, embracing life and death as one.

Persephone in the Pandemic
Elizabeth Woolfenden

As my bleeds spaced out, I found myself struggling in every single area of my life.

I was burnt out, overwhelmed and vulnerable.

I clung to nature like a life raft. at times, I was literally floored by my perimenopause and needed to lie on the earth for hours on end and watch the ants closely, like I did as a toddler, only this time they were transporting fallen pomegranate seeds.

I then became mesmerized by the pomegranates surrounding me here in Spain and I started spending my days amongst the pomegranate trees, eating them, playing with the jewel like seeds and photographing them, obsessively.

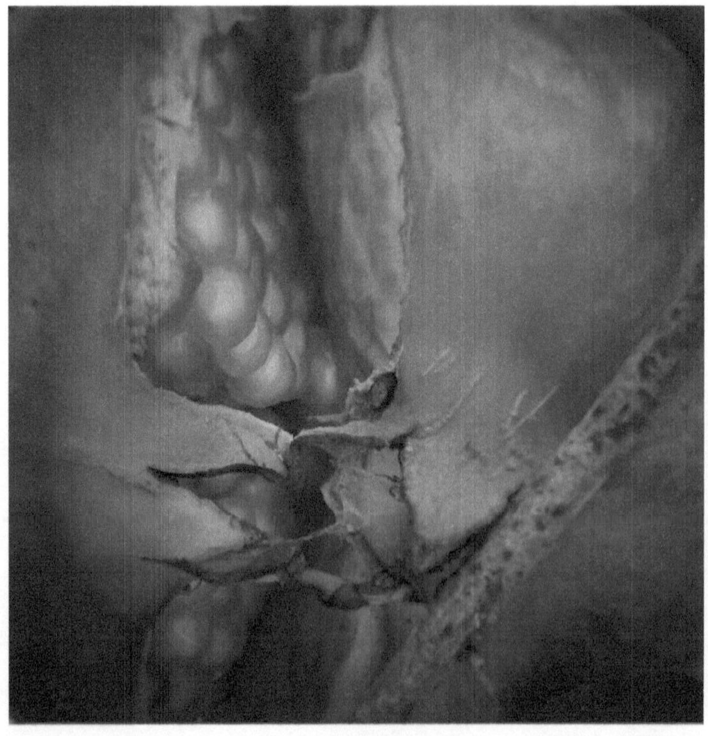

I have taken many hundreds of photos of pomegranates over the past 4 years.

Whilst this pomegranate obsession is still a bit of a mystery to me, I do see that it 'brought me to my senses'. I read over and over again the myth of Persephone and, when I found myself lying belly down on the earth, I would imagine that somehow my heart and soul was being opened and operated on by the technicians of the underworld

These deep and intricate operations woke me up to the fact that the 'too tight' life that I was living was beginning to smell deadly, something about my connection with these red seeds has enabled me to say 'No!', 'Stop!' and 'That is ENOUGH' and also more recently: 'THIS is who I am'
I delight in this.

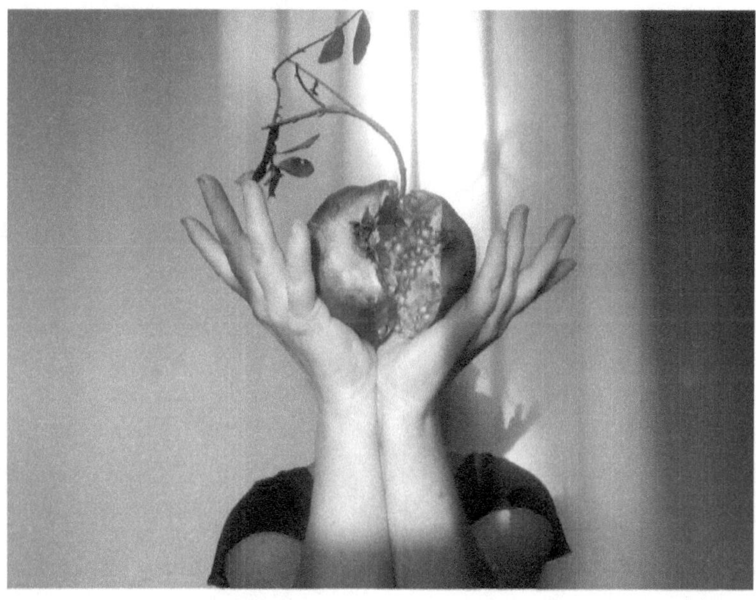

Honest Musings of a Crone
Suzanne Taylor-Torres

I have to say to you, as I sit here pondering my life, wandering through the passages of time... I am amazed! This gift of existence, this physical manifestation for soul education, is at its most sacred destination now. I am moving into the beginnings of "old-age."

I can now say I am a Crone. I am in the place of winter. The quiet time to reflect on the past, and settle into myself. The seeds of wisdom have been sown into me through the events of my life here on the earth plane. They allow me to sit with the Elders and impart my wisdoms.

Oh, how quickly did this happen! Yesterday's childhood, the springtime of my life, is fondly remembered. The endless hours spent outdoors swinging on my old wooden swing. Looking up into the tall oaks. Listening to their supple green leaves shuffling in the breeze. My young mind open to all the possibilities and innocent fantasies for the future.

Then, stepping into adulthood and growing into those possibilities. Blooming like summer to my life's work as a teacher, marriage, motherhood, and all the trials that went with these.

These challenges that watered those seeds of wisdom for my later years.

More and more of these seeds popping up in mid-life, as I began to reap what I had sown: divorces, remarriage, illness, home sales, moves, new employment... And the dreaded menopause, aged 55.

I did not mourn no longer being able to bear children. My motherhood experience was more than fulfilling. But, for a minute, I did mourn the loss of the ability to do so, noting that my body no longer flowed with reproductive sap. Instead, the beginning of withering was on the horizon. Perhaps you can relate. All one could do was stay healthy, eat properly, exercise, rest, and use lots of moisturizer.

My mind needed me to stay busy, until the day that ever-loving wisdom softened the dread and brought acceptance. Busy, busy, busy. Did I notice life was marching on? And so quickly? Did I realize the challenges, decisions, losses, gains, heartaches, and joys would all turn into each and every wrinkle I see on my face now? Ahh, seeds of wisdom!

So many years have gone by. The body is tired, the mind haunted by regrets. The heart is still healing from its wounds.

Do I need to continue reviewing the past? No, that time is over. Infinite wisdom tells me life is about joy, love, sharing, and enjoyment. It's about being in this world but not of it.

Harmonizing with love energy and moving within that and creating from that. The material things really don't matter. It's about being true to oneself, others and our word. It always was, but youth drives impatience, fear and uncertainty. Now I know, decisions no longer need to be made from those.

In my sixties, I am a young Elder. I have settled into myself, and can be confident in who I am and what I know. I choose to be on the wheel that is inside the wheel. While I may be in the winter of the life wheel, nature has provided an eternal wheel of the seasons where, after winter, spring begins anew. (And yes, even after menopause, one can still be productive and creative. Just in a different way.) Oh, I can see the projects now. I look forward to the new relationships and opportunities to serve. Especially with this accumulated treasure chest of knowledge.

Perhaps this spring, I shall buy a new swing to enjoy under the trees once again. Daydreaming and manifesting the rest of my future still here on the earth plane. You can do that too, my Sister.

After all, with all this Crone wisdom, it will be easier than ever. Amazing!

Memory Keeper
Lauren Raine

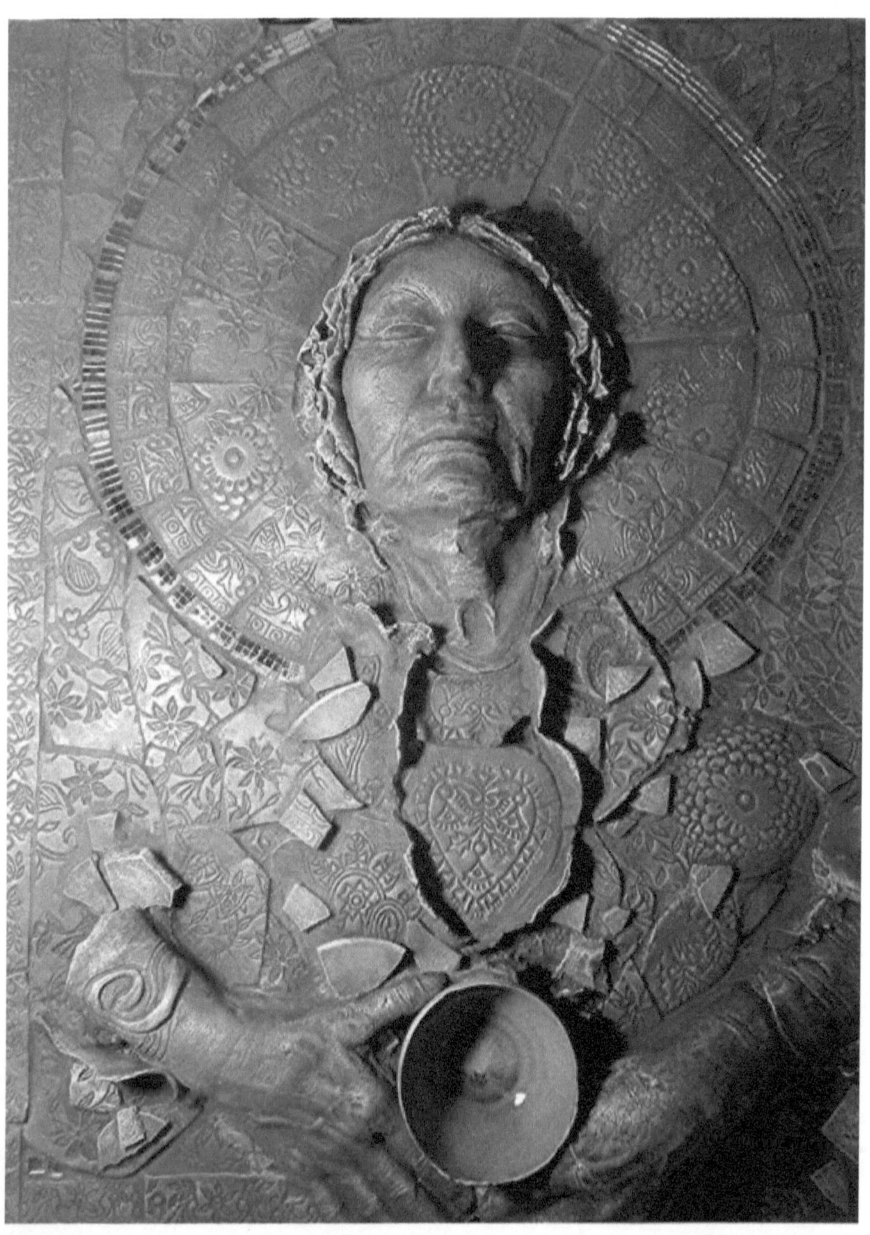

Romancing the Crone
Sue Lobo

In the cold cracked dawn I look into the mirror of my life &
ponder. I see wrinkles, lumps, bumps, saggy bits, all rather like the
etchings of the ancient tor, shaped through aeons by raging
storms & unforgiving suns.

Sagging breasts, having served their purpose, now at rest from
mewling babes & pawing, hungry men.

Varicose veins run like African rivers down the length of my tired
legs, reminding me that I am still alive.

I look down at my gnarled misshapen feet whom have taken me
through deserts, across oceans, roaming this earth in my seeking.
I look upon them as my travelling family, each toe a member,
related to each other by blood, sinew, tendon, always together.

Now these feet resembling roots, want to stay where they are, dig
into the earth & belong.

I feel the wild winds of winter in my hair of snow, soft & silver like
my mother Luna, the Moon.

I peer deep into my old, wise eyes, the delta from whence rivers
flowed with a myriad of joys, & many pains, now as arid as Kalahari
stones, windows of my history, where I see my past, my present, &
what's to come.

My voice is no longer the tinkling of spring bells, but now has the
melodic eloquence of the wailings of childbirth, & the songs of
lovers long gone.

I smile an old smile at what I see.

No Botox, lifting's, nips, tucks, & fillers for me, I am happy with who
I am.

Folk may ask, is this the rambling-be-petaled voice of consolation?
Sop to my sad befuddled ageing?

No, I am romancing the Crone,
the old Goddess,
embracing the woman she was, is, & will be,
thanking her for her wisdom to grow.

Self-Portrait – Mexico
Liliana Kleiner

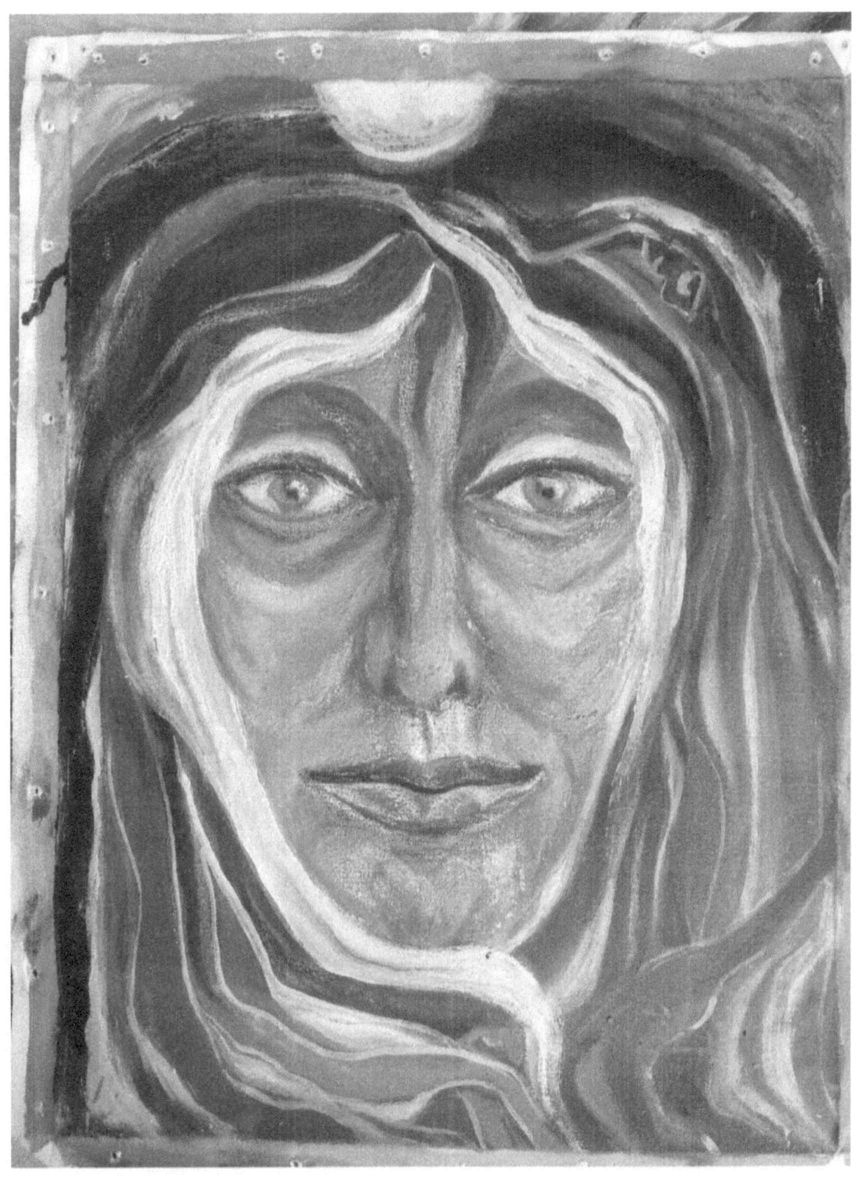

Creating a Meaningful Menopause
Jude Lally

Over and over, I felt the calling and I finally paid full attention through the unfolding of serendipity: a map falling out of a book, a place name mentioned on the radio and a stone, from a familiar beach, appearing on my desk. While I have visited the Scottish Hebridean Isle of Eigg before, it seems that previous visits were mere preparation for this visit.

Answering this call required a pilgrimage, a journey that took me on a four-hour train ride on the West Highland train line, which weaves through the spectacular scenery of Rannoch Moor and brings you into a realm of mountains. Even although it was May, there were still snow patches on the high peaks.

An hour ferry ride then marks a welcome threshold of leaving the mainland, facing west, and watching a small island grow bigger. The next day, as the sun slowly began its descent, saw me climbing up a steep path to visit the Loch of the Big Women. The Gaelic name of this island is the Isle of the Big Women.

The day was giving over into a long lingering twilight, a time in which the land is painted in a wash of its true colors. Faces normally obscured in daytime appear in the hillside and cliffs. Twilight is a time that's not quite day and not yet night, it is a place where magic resides.

I laughed to myself as I walked alone thinking that some people's idea of a holiday is to sun themselves on hot sandy beaches, and here was I heading up to a small loch instructed by a vision I had in an otherworldly journey.

On arriving at the loch, I was embraced by a rich silence, highlighted by the odd chirp of a bird, and a fish breaking the surface of the loch. The loch lies on a high point in the island and offers a wonderful view of the Isle of Skye and the dramatic peaks of the Isle of Rum. There is a small island in the middle of the loch, and it is said that the 'big women' lived on this little island.

When I think of these 'big women' I don't think of women of gigantic proportions, I think of women who were respected, were admired and looked up to. History seems to have forgotten exactly who the big women are, yet there are threads that remember islands ruled by women.

There is a story that when one of the early Irish monks, Saint Donnan came to the island in the 5th century, the local Queen of Moidart, a Pagan, was none too pleased. She sent her female warriors who demanded that Donnan and his followers come out of the church to face the warriors or else be slaughtered. Donnan replied that they would emerge once they had finished their mass, and as they did they were killed by the warriors.

That is not the end of the tale as it is said that that night strange glowing lights emanated from the slain bodies, and the warrior women followed, hypnotized. They took the same path up to the Loch as I had just walked but they didn't stop at the shore and followed the lights under the waves and drowned.

As I took off my rucksack and sat down it suddenly dawned on me that I wasn't alone. I could sense that there were figures of women lined up along the banks of the Loch.

I had the strongest feeling that I was here for a purpose, and that I was to submerge myself under the water. Even with an irrational fear of deep water, there was no second thinking, no debate or bargaining. I stripped off to a t-shirt, carefully waded out, for the sharp stones at the bottom of the loch were painful to walk on, until I was waist high in the loch.

I held my breath and ducked down under the surface of the water, I was barely under the water for a second or two, but it was as if time stood still. Even with my eyes shut I saw faces under the water; women's faces whose hair was floating around like reeds.

I emerged elated, as if I had swam underwater around the entire circumference of the loch. While women on the banks had vanished, I felt the full weight of this call, this initiation, yet it wasn't until the next year that I realized that this was my initiation into menopause, my beginning on the path of peri-menopause.

A Midwife

Reading Ursula Le Guin's essay sparked the idea that I needed a midwife for my menopausal journey. While she writes that within this journey a woman needs to give birth to herself, I wanted a guide for this birth. For my midwife, I chose the Cailleach as she and I have a long history. I know the storms she creates as she stomps through a landscape in an angry mood. I know the mists she veils the landscape and the mountains behind, days she doesn't want to have to deal with anyone or anything. I've been at the end of many a trick she has played, and I'm grateful to know her gentler moods when falling asleep on the hill in summer afternoons, then awaking to see a deer bound off. She and I have been in conversation before I started bleeding, and now I enter a different relationship with her after the bleeding has ceased.

As I journeyed deeper into menopause I began searching for stories, looking for rituals, for meaning within this rite of passage and for a community of women to share it all with, to hear their stories and listen to their experiences. At the same time, I began to create a midwife doll.

While I've made many Cailleach dolls, it was a special ritual to create a Cailleach doll as my midwife. I call myself a radical doll maker, following the tradition back to its roots, to hands that carved figures such as the menopausal Woman of Willendorf, and the stick and stone, fur and bone dolls that didn't survive. Dolls created for sacred rituals, to petition the Great Mother to bring favorable weather, for safety, for conception and for protection in birth and all the things we today petition the old ones for.

Dolls are curious creations as they hold a foot in this world and a foot in the otherworld. They hold stories and an invitation to listen and engage with that story. A doll is something to hold aspects of your story as you weave the threads of meaning together.

"Dolls serve as talismans. Talismans are reminders of what is left but not seen, what is so, but is not immediately obvious. The talismanic numen of the doll is that it reminds us, tells us, sees ahead for us. This intuitive function belongs to all women. It is a massive and fundamental receptivity. Not receptivity as once touted in classical psychology, that is a passive vessel. But receptivity as in possessing immediate access to a profound wisdom that reaches to women's very bones." –Clarissa Pinkola Estés

The Journey: Descent, Deep and the Return

Like the great mythic journeys, menopause as a rite of passage consisting of three parts: the descent, the deep and the return. The festivals of the dark of the year offer the perfect map for menopause. Autumn Equinox begins the descent while Samhain and Winter Solstice form the deep, Imbolc and Spring Equinox herald the return.

As menopause generally comes upon a woman in the autumn of her life, unless induced medically, it is the starting place for preparing for the journey.

The first stirrings of the descent of menopause are mirrored in autumn equinox. As harvests are gathered, we too can gather what we might need for the journey. A much-loved ritual for this time of year is lining a deep black cauldron with objects that represent the help and wisdom I might need and leaving space for the things I don't know I'll need.

The middle part of the journey, the deep, is mirrored in Samhain and the Winter Solstice. The deep of the journey is like the caterpillars breaking down within the pupae, letting go of old selves with faith that all we need will evolve within the new form. It's a shedding of past selves, much loved selves and so there can be a keening for our loss, but it's all part of the ritual.

We don't need to do any of this alone, for there is a place to go, a place we will be welcomed. The Cave of the Grandmothers is a place to be with wise elders.

At Samhain, the Cailleach makes her age-old journey to the whirlpool of Corryvrecken, the Cailleach's Cauldon. She washes her great plaid in the churning waters, uttering an ancient incantation. As she lifts it up and around her shoulders the last drops of water instantly freeze and dust the surrounding hills with the first dusting of winter snow. One winter role she carries out is in striking life down dead, returning it to its roots, for without death there can be no renewal of life in spring.

The churning waters of her cauldron can feel like menopause when we feel that change of identity, that breaking down, reforming and transformation. This isn't a place to fear for this is the liminal place, the in-between place, the threshold, and the place where the magic happens.

The sun is reborn at Winter Solstice and a ritual in acknowledging our rebirth is in considering who we wish to become? What is it you wish to accomplish in life? What knowledge or skills might you require? How do you share those skills with others?

The festivals of Imbolc and Spring Equinox mark the return phase. Imbolc is the festival of the Goddess Brighid, where she is welcomed back into the world. Winter still holds us in her grip, yet Brighid brings hope, a hint of things to come. Hers is an active hope, rooted in action, rather than just words.

Ritual can be inspired by Brighid's activism, through making plans. Hope needs action otherwise it ends up as wishful thinking.

Brighid is a threshold Goddess and one who is midwife of new souls coming into the world, yet she is also there at the end of life when souls leave this world to return to the Otherworld. She can be a midwife to us in this holy threshold rite of the journey to becoming crone.

Spring Equinox is the great return; it symbolizes arriving on the other side, post menopause. There is a ritual in seeing who it is that extends a hand, who aids our return. It is a point to review the journey and begin to put our plans into action and put new insights to work.

Creating a meaningful menopause is a radical act in today's world, honoring this rite of passage with ritual and ceremony. Telling our story is to give it meaning and make menopause matter, as we become our own big women and evoke even bigger and wilder hags. The Wheel of the Year is a path we can journey through the descent, the deep and the eventual return, the breaking down and being reborn.

References:

Dressler, Camille. 1998. Eigg. *The Story of An Island*. Polygon, Edinburgh, UK.

Estés, Clarissa Pinkola. 1992. Women Who Run With the Wolves. Myths and Stories of the Wild Woman Archetype. Ballantine Books, New York, US. Pg 91.

Le Guin, Ursula. "The Space Crone." *Women of the 14th Moon. Writings on Menopause.* The Crossing Press, CA, USA. Taylor, D and Sumrall, Amber Coverdale (Eds). 1991.

My Cailleach Midwife Doll
Jude Lally

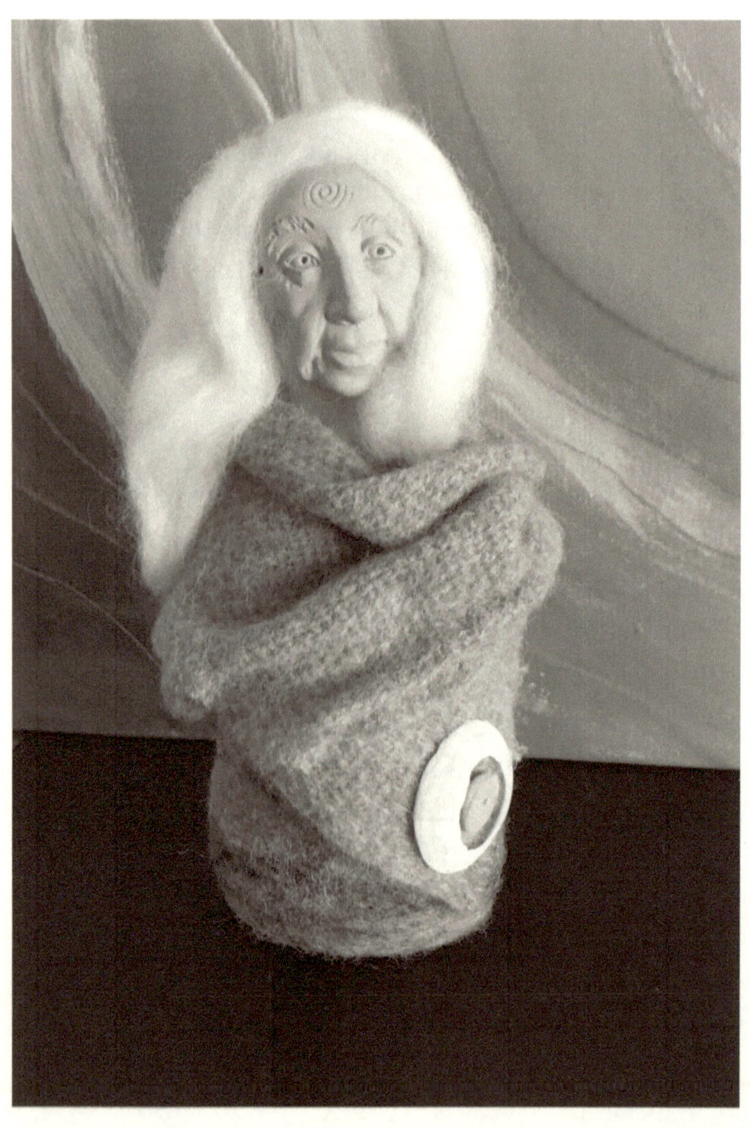

Invitation to Live
Karen Storminger

When I was young,
They said,

"You're too fat."
So I starved myself

"Your laugh is too loud."
So I quieted my joy

"You're too bossy."
So I stepped back behind others

"You're too smart."
So I hid my thoughts

"You're expecting too much." So I walked away...
And I made myself small

And the years passed by
And Silver strands began to weave through my head
And I heard the whispers on the wind
Then, Goddess said,
"You are as I made you"
So I Nourished my body and soul
"Let me hear your voice."
So I Let loose my joy
"I need leaders to do my work"
So I Stepped forward and Took charge of my life...

"Women of wisdom change the world."
So I Spoke my mind

"I expect much of you"
So I accepted her invitation, and began to live

A Crone's Prayer
Karen Storminger

Blood and bone Sinew and joint
Hands that held mine, once held by another
I honor my Ancestors all from one Mother
Grandmother, Old Crone, Wise Woman,
you who guards souls at their end
My elders have met thee
Ancestors now gone beyond
Watching over our lives from beginning to end
As my hand holds another, the next in our line
I know that one day
Your hand will find mine

Menopause Remodel

Trista Hendren

Peri-menopause is a deep initiation to our highest selves—which often means we have to burn shit to the ground.

As we were wrapping this anthology up, we began a major remodel of our basement. We initially thought we would have to replace all the flooring—and possibly tear down some walls. But as we began the work, and peeled layer after layer of faulty remodeling attempts from a century of previous owners, we realized that much of the foundation and walls were completely rotten.

The air quality where we had slept the past 4 years could not have been good for us. Our bedroom was slowly poisoning us.

Everything had to be removed. We had to rebuild absolutely everything from the ground up.

It occurred to me that this is very much like my own peri-menopause initiation.

The foundation of my life was built on patriarchal dysfunction. I coped and adapted the best I could for 47 years. But at the root of my beliefs about my own worth, everything was rotten. I had to step outside of those patternings to reclaim my Divine essence.

I have been torn apart, and have put myself back together, many times throughout my life—but I realize now I may have kept some of the old wallpaper up to save myself some steps.

The Crone Initiation can be brutal. She reveals everything that needs to go. And She's not "nice" or patient about it!

There is nothing quite like seeing the entire bottom floor of your house in your own front yard. The rot had been hidden from sight for 4 years under dozens of paint jobs, wallpaper layers and old floorings. We spent many evenings around a huge bonfire in our front yard. I felt ecstatic burning all the old shit—and even better when Anders took what could not safely be burned to the dump.

Peri-menopause is my opportunity to remodel my life from the foundation. Ripping down walls is noisy. There's drilling, sawing, throwing wood to the ground, and then a filthy mess to clean-up. My home is 100 years old—and we literally had soggy wood at the foundation that Anders had to pull up by the handful.

We have at least 5,000 years of patriarchal conditioning to remove—it is going to get messy at times.

Even amongst the chaos, I could feel the energy shifting as we got rid of the gunk. The air quality became cleaner, and we became healthier. It will take at least 3 times longer to do everything right, but now that we have seen what lies beneath the facade, there is no other way.

The Crone offers us an invitation: It is up to us to accept or decline it. Either we walk in Her beauty and truth—or we keep plastering over faded wallpaper and rehashing old shit.

While I have many decades before I can claim the crown of the Crone, I am excited about the process of becoming a glorious Hag.

The Power of the Crone
Arna Baartz

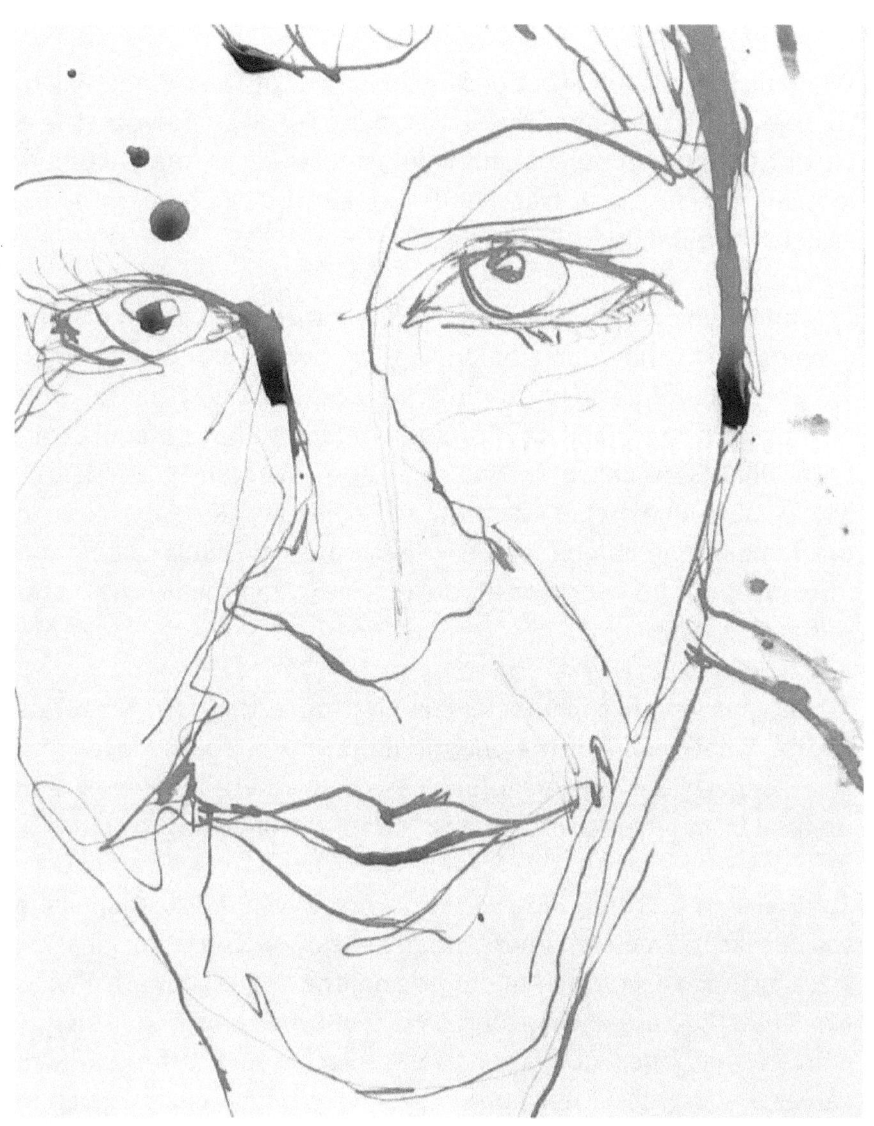

A Visit With The Crone. She Has Been With You All Your Life

Dale Allen

When discussing and experiencing the power of The Crone, I like to come through the lens of the archetypes. Like all archetypes, She is part of the human psyche and belongs to all of us: men, women, lesbian, gay, bisexual, transgender, queer, questioning, intersex, asexual, non-Binary – all humans.

The archetypes are without boundary – they're like dreams and imagination – they don't belong to solely one group or gender. They are unbounded. For example, we wouldn't say, "That can only be imagined by a man." Or, "Only a woman can have that dream." I like what Gary Bobroff writes. He says, "Women often identify with a masculine archetypal form and men may see themselves in the feminine archetypal stories. There are no *shoulds* being put forward about how someone is best to live (other than with greater self-awareness)."

Archetypes are like characters in literature. F Scott Fitzgerald wrote: "That is part of the beauty of literature. You discover that your longings are universal longings, that you're not lonely and isolated from anyone. You belong."" Yes, we all belong.

To discuss the Crone, I invite you to come into a dream space, a space that is timeless, where creativity flows, where imagination gives birth to reality. Within our psyche, the archetypes are always available, they are always there. We just tend to align our energy with certain ones at certain times. Archetypes offer us such valuable insight... They offer pathways and perspective to understand where we are in life. They bring us richness and meaning – taking us out of the mundane, connecting us to healthy inner power, passion, and purpose.

Swiss psychiatrist Carl Jung described archetypes as models of people, behaviors, or personalities. For Jung, the psyche was composed of three components: the ego, the personal unconscious, and the collective unconscious. The collective unconscious is where the archetypes exist. These models are unlearned; they are innate, universal, and hereditary. An archetype is an inward image in the human psyche that exerts a powerful influence on the nature of an individual personality and in turn on the larger culture.

So, the Crone or Wise Woman is one of many archetypes. But, She's not well understood…. In many ways her value has been lost to us. Her ancient power has been reduced to characterization as the evil, ugly witch. Our culture so prizes youth and productivity, sending a clear signal to fear anything to do with age and elder years. And, we surely have a deficit in psychic guidance around mortality.

So, we may look at the Crone and say, "I don't think I want to get to know her!" But she exists and has existed in us since the day we were born. And she's so powerful! She is a Keeper of Wisdom. One of her great teachings is that… Life is a progression of disappearances. Life goes something like this: you build it, you structure it, you count on it, you think you've arrived somewhere, but at some point, you realize the impermanence of things – the process starts again. Yet, there are certain threads that remain, threads that connect to our Inner Core, which is constant and timeless. And that Inner Core is what we need to connect to, because if we don't, when the things we constructed in life aren't the endpoint we imagined, or if things come crashing down, we can get lost in painful shambles.

Winter provides a great metaphor to explore the Crone. The winter landscape offers us its barrenness. You don't see the fruits and the flowers. You don't see all of your creations. You don't see the garlands, the Maypole. You don't see anything but that bleak, white landscape and the trees silhouetted against the sky. You come to such a barren landscape in your life when your what you've constructed has fallen. And this can happen at any point in life – for example, when you graduate high school. Adults forget and will say, "Oh… Their whole lives are ahead of them!" But, if you recall, that's a time of a kind of death. Deaths happen even during childhood as we progress from one stage to another.

These deaths happen throughout life. You get to a point where – what you put your efforts into – your plans, your dreams, your hopes – the ways that you came to define yourself and your life, fall. And you find yourself asking, "What happened? I'm standing here now, and I can't see any of it anymore. I don't know where to go. I can't see the path; it's covered with snow. I don't know anything here. It's very still. It's very silent." What was familiar is gone. We can't fast-forward to Spring. In fact, if we try to fast-forward to something that will immediately fill the void, we will likely find that it is false, and it will fall. If we have the courage to stand in the stillness and simply look around us, there's an invitation that occurs. It's an invitation to take us deep down within ourselves.

Within you is your own Wise Woman Crone who has given you Her strength and guidance all your life. Imagine now that you have been walking in a winter landscape. No path is visible in the snow. You come upon a cave lit by the glow of a small fire. You are drawn in by a warm and very welcoming energy. You see that the fire is tended by a very Ancient Woman. When Her eyes meet yours, you see that She is also ageless, timeless. There is something so very kind and deeply familiar about Her. She smiles and beckons you to sit beside her in the warm glow.

The CRONE Speaks:
"Welcome my dear, dear One. I am the Crone. I am the Winter. I am the stillness. I am the drawing inward. Look to me. I am the Winters on your journey. I am not boisterous with newness and growth. I am not the grand flower festivals of your life or the overflowing harvest of your efforts. In me are the many deaths of your days, for nothing can grow if it does not shed what must die.

And you carry so much that has finished its purpose...

It is hard to let go, but would you reject me? Would you make all efforts to eternally produce in a great show of fruits and flowers? It is a hollow pursuit, for the field must lay still under the snows of winter – fallow some years even as the seasons change, in order to be replenished for sowing. Look to me. I am that part of you that in wisdom allows the deaths to come, that reveals the folly of your ever clinging to the familiar but confining. I am below the surface, deep down in darkness beneath the harsh and bleak winter landscape. Look to me and do not be deceived – for under the cold, cold snow lies your truth, your vitality, your destiny, your soul.

It is I who beneath the frozen ground cradles the seeds of your innocence. It is I who in time unfolding encourages the seeds to sprout. It is I who brings forth the bloom of your destiny.

Do you remember the days of your youth? Do you remember your innocence as in your inward-sense. The unencumbered Beingness of your Authentic Self? The spark of your knowing that you have place in this world? For some it was years in childhood of knowing. For some, one precious summer. For others a knowing that came through in a flash, in spite of outer circumstances. But you knew that you had a place and a purpose. I tell you this innocence is not a time of life that passes; it is a vital force that must be tended and kept alive.

Would you let the flame of your innocence go out? Every inauthentic role you take on and refuse to let go of dims the light from view. Every time you imprison yourself, claiming that you must serve others. Every time you refuse to act on your own behalf, you shut away the light – closed the door on the child, on your innocence.

Here in the darkness, deep within the earth, in the embrace of a silent cave, I tend this vital flame. You must know me to really know this fire. I am all of your experience. I am every failed effort, every seeming mistake, every disappointment, every rejected aspect of yourself… I am every triumph. I am every realization of what matters most in Life. I am here and whole and over-brimming with love for all of it

Look to me. Know me. Do not dance on the edges of your life, fearfully holding fast to your safe havens of comfort – your self-definitions. You hold fast to that part of yourself that has a clever answer, an acceptable plan, a safe pattern to follow, a way to avoid letting go of that which must go. Having created this facsimile of yourself, you guard it, believing that it will keep you from the changing seasons. This veneer of yours is paper-thin. With its clever answers – it's busy-ness – it attempts scurry away from winter. But your paper-thin veneers fall like the autumn leaves off the trees. It is no matter. Your roots run so deep, right down to me.

Come into the darkness. Come into the night. Come into the stillness. Brave the cold and the wind and come to the cave. Enter and go deep inside. Come into that part of yourself that has no clever answers, that does not know – that only knows that the veneer you made will not sustain you, and that somewhere, somewhere there is a small flame to tend.

Come to me deep beneath the snows, down inside the cave. I wait within, tending, tending the flame. Let that which must go, go. Take courage. You do not need answers now. Take courage in not knowing. Take courage in not doing.

Come sit beside me. Come sit beside the fire. It is all you need in this moment. Feel the warmth and peace.

I am here always, and this flame I tend is within you always. The spring will come again; it is not your doing.

And in the spring, as you move into the world, it is in full alignment with your soul – it is You taking Your place in the world. For you are ever innocent and true and your experience is precious.

You will sprout up as surely as a green shoot from the black earth, pushing up past the debris. The paper-thin veneers you had left behind are scattered around you like fallen leaves – the very fodder that becomes the rich soil that nurtures you. The spring always comes, and when it comes, it is you that blooms."

I believe that the metaphor of standing uncertain in a winter landscape, whether it's still falling snow and a pathway you can't see, or whether it's a great howling wind of a blizzard, this winter landscaped calls us to turn inward into the stillness within.

It's a metaphor for the collective right now. Collectively, we just don't know what's going to happen, where we're all headed... in a more pronounced way at this time. We suspect that something new wants to be born. In the wisdom of the feminine tradition, it must be: Birth, growth, death, renewal. The birth, the new beginning, the new reality cannot come until the death comes.

It's an ever-turning circle. Every one of us holds a seed to what wants to emerge. When we are in alignment, when we go right to the Core to our authentic selves, there's something in us that wants to come out, that is part of the world as it is being reborn.

Every one of us holds a seed as co-creators of this new reality that's emerging. The only way that we can do this, is if we are all willing to regularly access that space of inward stillness... to make peace with the unknowing, though it can be tough to do. It is where the seat of the new is being nurtured.

We are all in this together – we all share this moment on the planet – even that is just amazing to ponder... In all of time on this earth, we all happen to be here in this moment together – in this profoundly important experience of all of us creating a new reality together. You count. You matter. You are critical to what wants to be created. Know that and know it well. Trust the light of the Crone's fire. Stay in the stillness and together we will emerge in the dawn of new beginnings.

I Bow (Crone Version)
Arlene Bailey

I have stopped apologizing for myself

Stopped wiping the dripping blood
just to make myself socially acceptable
to the masses

Stopped apologizing for old woman's body
With sagging tits and rounded belly

Hair that now mirrors the moon
And my trusty walking stick gifted
By Grandmother Oak

For I am still...

A wild woman and I own
Every
Single
Cell
In
This
Aging
Morphing into Willendorf
Called by the Morrighan
And Erishkigal
Body

I am still...

The Wolf prowling under the Full
Moon sky, both loner and tribal

The Tiger stalking her prey knowing
She has the key to removing their bindings

The Panther lying seductively in wait
for just the right moment to pounce

The Owl in flight under the Dark Moon
diving towards the deepest depths of the
Dark underworld with eyes to see in the
dark and wings to soar to the highest light

AND

I am still...

Virgin, Seductress and Mother

Amazon and Warrioress

Sorceress, Witch and Conjure Woman

Medial Woman and Keeper of Realms

Modern woman and Ancient one

AND

I AM...

Grandmother Turtle moving at her own pace
knowing she has existed lifetimes upon lifetimes
and will exist for that many more for the codes
of the universe are written upon her very skin

I AM...

The Old Antlered One who has walked
the Ley Lines, the Dragon Lines
since before time was time

I AM...

SHE who exists in the last stages of life
SHE who sees through the Veil, Winter Woman
Dark Mother and Bringer of Death Mysteries

I AM CRONE!

ALL connected by the blood of ancestors
and woman's shared experience
through millennia

I am all these things and more
and I will NOT apologize for the scars
and wounds that brought me to this place
This NOW of owning it all
regardless of the opinions of others
or the stakes of a society that would
see me in chains or even dead

I will not apologize for the strength found and the wisdom honed
through rituals studies, teachings and inner world knowings

I will not apologize for standing strong
in the face of untenable atrocities

I am a Sovereign Being
Walking this Earth as Old Woman,
Crone, Hag, Dark Mother, Death Mother
Even Death Herself
Again and again and again

Through all the Timelines and
Lifetimes after Lifetimes
Feral

Wild
and Free

I am Crone

AND

I Bow To Me

I Bow (Crone Version), Arlene Bailey ©2022

Spider Woman

Lauren Raine

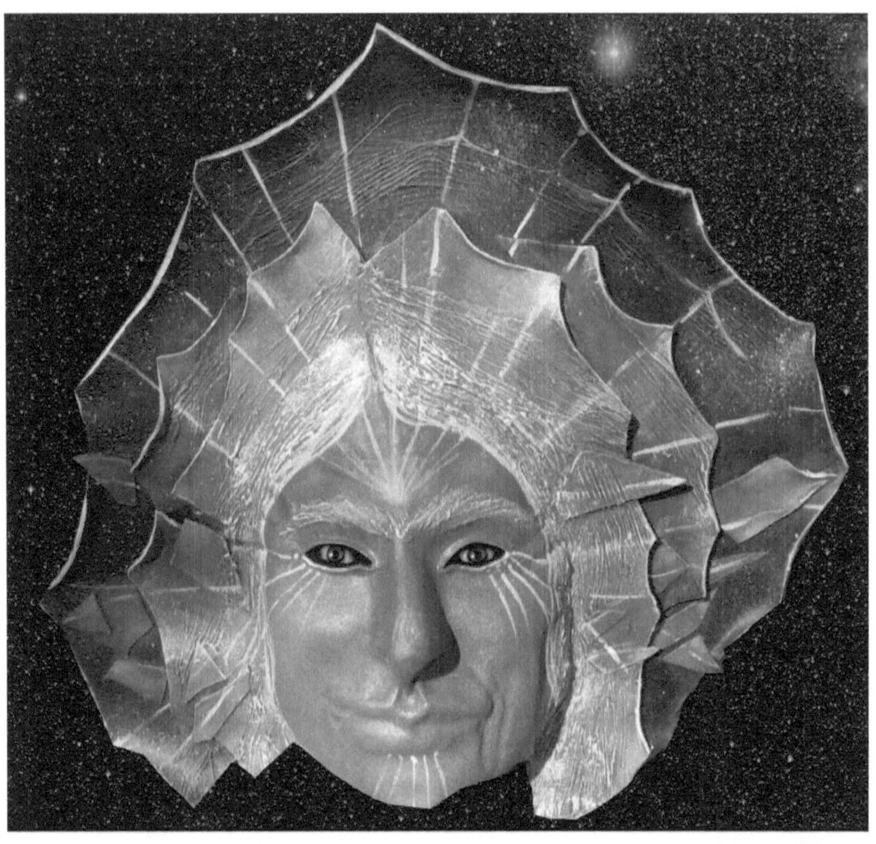

The Ash Grove

H. Byron Ballard

I claimed my own cronehood the January that the covid pandemic took hold. I could have claimed it several years earlier, but I didn't feel ready. In December several friends and family members died unexpectedly, and my world felt both smaller and deeper. I chose to do a private ritual and to refocus my work, as my dreams were filled with visions of different, older worlds. This is one of those Crone-World dreams.

The ash grove, how graceful, how plainly tis speaking
The wind through it playing has language for me;
When o'er the light through its branches is breaking,
A host of kind faces is gazing on me,
The friends of the childhood again are before me.
Fond memories waken as freely I roam.
With soft whispers laden its leaves rustle o'er me,
The ash grove, the ash grove alone is my home.
My laughter is over, my step loses lightness,
Old countryside measures steal soft on my ears;
I only remember the past and its brightness,
The dear ones I mourn for again gather here.
From out of the shadows their loving looks greet me,
And wistfully searching the leafy green dome,
I find other faces fond bending to greet me,
The ash grove, the ash grove alone is my home.
Welsh, traditional

A yew tree stands as a sort of sentinel beside an overgrown trail, a path that wends into the old and ragged forest. The wood has stood at the edge of the wheat field for as long as anyone can remember, and the thin path grows thinner with each passing harvest-tide.

Not many are brave enough to wander into the wood and most only do so in daylight, in order to track down a wayward sheep or equally wayward child.

There is only one group of people who tread that path and those are the old women of the village. The healers and wise women. The grannies and child-watchers. The crones. The wynd widens for their slow and steady feet, the branches on either side seem to fold onto themselves when the dark Moon rises unseen, and the crones walk. They leave the supper on the table and comfort the little ones with sweet meats and dollies. Each bends to pick up her market basket filled with bread, herbs, homebrewed beer. The adult children shake their heads and fret about the weather, about wolves, about highwaymen out on the roads after sunfall. But the old women only shake their heads and touch their cheeks for a soft kiss from their offspring. There is work to be done and it is the sort of work that only the crones may do, that only crones can do.

Their number changes every year, like the path in the wood. The eldest of the elders pass through the thin veil and join their before-mothers in the lands of the dead. Spry, younger crones join the circle of old women to learn their ways and keep their wisdom. One day they will be the eldest and will walk through to join the before-mothers but not now. Now they are the youngest of the old and they swap baskets with the frailer women and offer their arms as extra support.

The women dress sensibly for the weather, wool cloaks in the gales of winter, soft shawls for summer nights. Hats in the rain, hair loose and flower-bedecked in the joy of late spring. They always have stout and sensible shoes no matter the season for the path into the wood can be unfriendly and prone to snagging the unwary.

At sunfall, they gather in the field and praise the soil that produces such a splendid crop. They sing to the spirits of the farmland and offer them the same sweet meats they gave the children. One very old woman uses her walking stick to pound the ground in a rhythmic massage of the dear and generous earth. Her sisters stamp their feet and there is a dance of sorts, in honor of the field and its soil. They are dancing it to sleep at the end of the growing year and dancing it awake in the early spring. The people of the village are allowed to watch from the other side of the field but are not allowed to join in or to come close. This would disturb the oldest magic, a magic in which they may not take part, not until they are old.

When the dark begins to creep out of the wood and into the neighboring fields, the crones pick up the baskets that were set down for the blessing dance and they move to the path's beginning. One by one and sometimes two by two, they step into the wood. It is then that the village turns away out of respect or superstition—who can say?

They don't see the lights that seem to grow from the earth to brighten the path before the old feet. They don't see the way the women straighten their backs and how their steps grow lighter, even the eldest of the elders. The crones move at a stately pace like elves trooping through the wood. They observe the eyes that watch from the undergrowth and the nightsounds of birds settling into the branches above them. A fox kit will sometimes dash between them, and its mother follows, swift and silent, to fetch the trickster back to the safety of the den beneath the bramblehedge. The crones laugh softly remembering their time as mothers, keeping the little ones as safe as could be, as warm and well-fed as the little kit and her sisters.

They walk, pacing like warhorses, for more than a mile. They aren't in a rush for they have the night ahead of them. The dark Moon is the Crone Moon, too, made for their work. Enough time to walk in and to walk out, enough time to do the work they are called to do.

There is always enough time for the ash grove, and the yew waits for their return with patience.

The wood is quiet now and the crones' journey almost complete. The path widens and the soft light that has accompanied them thus far begins to fade. Just ahead is the grove and it gleams with its own brightness, even on this night of no Moon. A carpet of mushroom and toadstools gives the grove this gleam, this radiance. The crones come to stand in the circle of the great ash trees, the rowans of memory and folktale. The trees rise far above the wise heads of the crones, their wisdom more vast and deeper than any human can imagine. The women set down their baskets and honor the sacred grove with three songs, sung one after the other, songs older than the women, older even than the trees. The women sing words that are not the words they speak at home and in the village. This is not the language of their family or of their people. It is an old tongue dark with history, with longing, with wrenching pain, with revelation. One after another, they sing each song three times and by the third time the new women know the old words and the chanting tunes. Three times three and the holy rite is done, the trees satisfied. The crones find seats amongst the trunks of the trees, and they settle in for the sharing, for the feasting, for the working.

The women pull hefty balls of woolen yarn from the baskets, along with smooth sticks, each topped with a fat bead and sharpened to a dull point at the other end. As they talk, they commence knitting, the wooden needles clacking as their fingers move. First there is gossip: stories about the babies and husbands, about handfastings and funerals, about newcomers to the village and the families who have left for the city.

The knitting is very fast, magically swift, flowing over their knees and onto the forest floor. Soon they attach the ends of each piece to the ends of the pieces on either side of them. Together they knit the edges and raise the long and complete circle over their heads, sounding their joy in the beauty of it with a loud, eerie cry. They drape the shawl over their shoulders and sit in the circle of its warmth and power.

The talk turns to other matters then, and we will not speak of that here. This is the careful deliberation that happens before any working can begin. These subjects are wide as the sky, higher than the western mountains and deeper than the well of Night that stands near the burying ground. The crones' voices are low now, almost whispers, but each word is clear as larksong. At last no words are spoken and the debate continues in spirit form, nothing to hear in the silent circle of old shawled women.

When the work and the method are at last agreed upon, the women's heads nod in unison, three times three, and they become impossibly still as though turned to rock. The ground in the rowan grove shimmers and the trees sway gently. The light grows brighter and the crones close their eyes, calling the power of the living soil into their working. They begin a new song, a song of sleet and lightning, of earthquake and landslide, even as their bodies remain preternaturally still. It is in the same harsh and haunted tongue as before and it rises and falls over and over and if one was counting the rising and the falling, we would find the crones' sacred triplets, three times three.

With each rise and fall, the sound expands to fill the grove and then the wood, flowing like wildfire into the village where the mothers sing lullabies to the children, holding them in the crook of their arms so they don't hear. Animals in the barns and pastures raise their heads and join in the rising and the falling, adding grunts and mooing, and the strained calls of the excited sheep. No one, not even the sleepy children, is afraid of the sound. It is cronesong, as usual and commonplace as the growl of the farm dog or the hiss of the watchful geese. Cronesong brings healing and luck, and everything good. It is said that when there is no more cronesong the world will grieve and mourn, and die at last, in cold silence.

The ash grove seems to spin, the trees wild in forceful winds. The women stand and open their eyes, and the light and the wind cease with the sound. The work is finished at last and the land, children and nervous sheep go back to sleep.

Hungry as hunters, the women open the baskets and share the food—bread and cheese, potted meats and dark beer. The gossiping tales return and there is so much laughter, as the crones refresh their bellies and wet their parched throats. Libation is poured for the trees and the soil. Crusts of bread and rinds of fruit are left for the birds and animals. The black of the eastern sky is giving way to grey and blue, and the sun's dawning.

The crones let the circle of wool fall to the ground, an offering to the night and the greenwood. They take up their empty baskets and make their way out of the grove, and down the path where they emerge from the old wood in the shadows of the yew. The sun is up now and the work of this dark Moon complete.

They kiss and embrace and turn their faces to the new day, and home.

Crone Wisdom
Judith Murphy

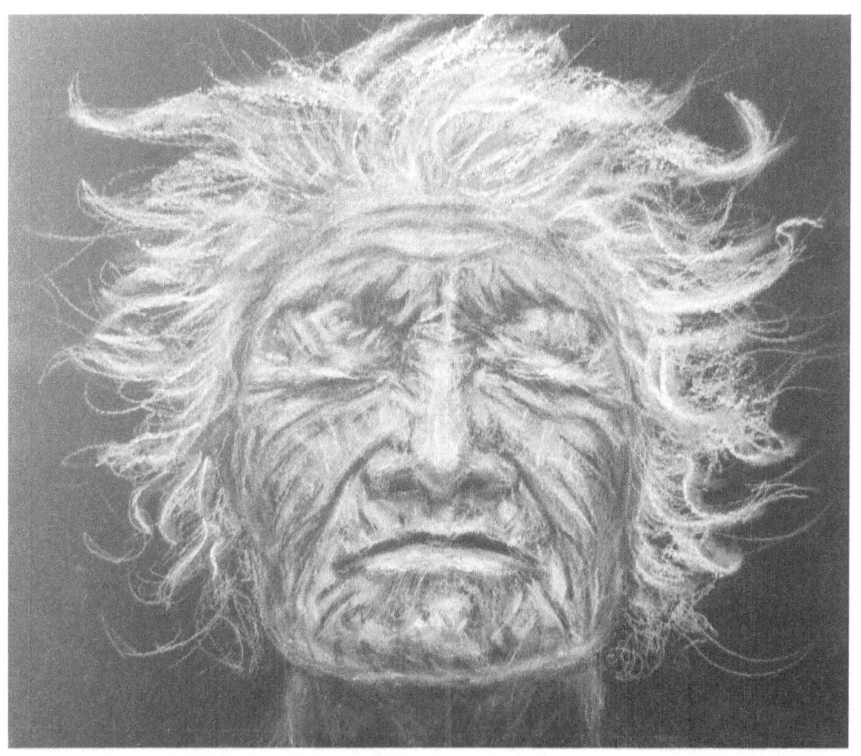

Crone's Return
Kay Louise Aldred

Can you feel Crone's Return?
Its bubbling, swirling. On the boil.
Women's Wisdom uncoupling from silence.
Hag is calling. Mighty staff in hand. Pounding the Earth.

Which now quakes and shakes with her rhythmic insistence.
The power of the Ancient is reclaiming its place.
The symphony completed. Feminine synergy.
The wielding Axe from the battle won.

Laughing witches gathering again in circle,
Reinstate the visibility of Medicine Women
As integral to community's thriving.
The position of Elder is understood and revered once more.

A great cleansing of the collective is underway,
The disinfecting rage of the Dark Goddess Woman
Eradicates pathogenic patriarchal thought forms and
Heals our womb from the pus of patriarchal infection.

As her ferocity replaces meekness and people-pleasing passes
As she takes up space. We take up space.
Biddy is back.
Interfering with clear intent.

Freedom. Pleasure. Embodiment.
Sovereignty. Self-Leadership.
Thriving Earth.

List of Contributors

Andrea Redmond has been a feminist rights activist, artist and pagan for over 50 years. She has been a devotee of The Morrigan since a young girl.

She was born on Prince Edward Island, Canada of Irish descent and moved to Ireland with her young family and there, she was one the first women in Belfast to paint wall murals. Her first mural in 1983 honoured women rights activists from Ireland, and South Africa. She has painted over 40 murals with similar themes and her work has featured in a number of publications and films on Northern Ireland.

She has worked and chaired a number of women's, art and multicultural groups. She has taught programs in art, community development and youth work. She is a mother to three children and returned to education in her 40s, completing her PhD, at the University of Ulster.

Andrea currently resides in rural Donegal, Ireland where she operates her art studio/workshop. Her artwork is in permanent collections and galleries in Ireland, Canada and the United States.

Angie Litvinoff is a Rites of Passage Guide for Midlife Women, a Modern Medicine Woman and an Artist. She helps women to find their joy, birth their true selves and awaken their midlife power.

She does this with RISE, her potent rites of passage ceremony immersion, working with processes, cycles, elements and the Goddess archetypes. Shares her own passion and self-expression through her Shamanic Goddess art. She has worked with 100s of women in the last 25 years to reconnect to their essence of soul and change their lives. Her message is simple, honour, create and express who you are and find your joy. To find out more see www.angielitvinoff.com.

Annie Finch is a poet, performer, and teacher. She is the author of a dozen books, including *The Poetry Witch Little Book of Spells, Eve, A Poet's Craft*, and the epic poem on abortion *Among the Goddesses*, which received the Sarasvati Award from ASWM. Her eight edited books include *Choice Words: Writers on Abortion,* the first major literary anthology on abortion. She holds a Ph.D. from Stanford University and descends from witches imprisoned in the Salem Witch Trials. Annie has taught widely and performs through Poetry Witch Ritual Theater.

She teaches classes in poetry, meter, witchery, and her original transformative teaching, The Magic of Rhythmically Writing, at PoetryWitchCommunity.org. You can find Annie on Twitter: @poetrywitch and Instagram: @thepoetrywitch.

Arlene Bailey is a visionary artist and author working in the realm of the Sacred Female in all her many visages. Arlene's paintings and poetry/prose reflect the raw, visceral and sacred wild in all women, while challenging and questioning everything we know to be true about the who of who we are as women walking in this time.

Through her magical weavings in word and paint—and, drawing on her trainings and skills as an Ordained Priestess, Women's Mysteries Facilitator, Wise Woman Herbalist, Energy Medicine Practitioner and Retired Anthropologist—Arlene invites women to step into personal sovereignty as they listen to their ancient memories and voice of their soul.

Published in several Girl God Books' anthologies, Arlene is also a monthly contributor to Return to Mago E-Magazine and has writings in two forthcoming Mago anthologies. Her work can also be found on The Sacred Wild, a page on Facebook about re- wilding woman's soul. Along with her partner and five cats, this Wild Crone lives on 18 acres of deep woods and quartz outcroppings in the Uwharrie Mountains of North Carolina, USA. www.facebook.com/sacredwildstudio www.instagram.com/arlenebaileyartist www.magobooks.com www.magoism.net

Arna Baartz is an artist, writer, educator and poet. She has been finger-painting from the beginning when her father, also creative, encouraged her by taping paper to the walls of their home and letting her loose with paint. As a result, she is an expressive artist with a belief in non-judgement, often purposely leaving her 'mistakes' in an attempt to allow the unfolding to participate in a finished piece. Arna influenced by her mother's creative story telling, also enjoys stringing words together to create a feeling. Poetry and writing fill many secret corners of her colourful life.

Her arts practice ranges in extremes from the creation of small and playful to large and serious. Most of Arna's work is an extension of her philosophical nature, bringing her gifts of personal insight and joy. Arna has won and been selected for many art awards including those of prestige and has had both art and words published extensively around the globe. Her first and favourite claim to fame however, was being held upside down and used as a paintbrush by Australian Artist, John Olsen. This fun was had at a workshop in St. John's Cathedral, Brisbane, 1973. Her writing and poetry has also been published throughout the world in a plethora of magazines and online forums.

Arna is delighted to have the opportunity to create in this lifetime. Her art, words and poetry are transcendental to a degree and offer the intention of unconditional love and hopefully a little dab of inspiration to anyone else on a similar journey. Arna's more recent publications include *New Love - a reprogramming toolbox for undoing the knots* (co-authored with Trista Hendren), *My Abundant Universe, The Creative Warrior, The Animals Know it* and *The Sun is in my Mouth*.

Her website is https://arnabaartz.com.au.

Barbara O'Meara, professional visual artist, art activist, published writer & co-editor of 'Soul Seers Irish Anthology of Celtic Shamanism'. Her 20 Solo Exhibitions include 'B.O.R.N. Babies of Ravaged Nations'. International juried shows include ASWM 'Wisdom Across the Ages', Lockhart Gallery New York 'Contemporary Irish Art' & Herstory 'Brigid's of the World' & 'Black

Lives Matter'. Community Arts include 'Stitched With Love' Tuam Baby Blanket laid out onsite at the Mother & Child Institution by survivors and families, at KOLO International Women's Non Killing Cross Borders Summit in Sarajevo and held by Bosnian women war survivors. 'Sort Our Smears' Campaign at 'Festival of FeminismS'. 'Home Words Bound' publication with National Collective of Community Based Women's Networks where her paintings accompany writing by Irish women about the Pandemic.

She is continually developing empowering women's 'Art as Activism' projects. She is honored to be featured in several Girl God Books and is the featured artist in a new publication, *My Name is Brigid* which launched on Brigid's Day 2022.

www.barbaraomearaartist.com

H. Byron Ballard, BA, MFA, is a western NC native, teacher, folklorist and writer. She has served as a featured speaker and teacher at Sacred Space Conference, Summerland Spirit Festival, Pagan Spirit Gathering, Southeast Wise Women's Herbal Conference, Glastonbury Goddess Conference, Heartland, Sirius Rising, Starwood, Scottish Pagan Federation Conference and other gatherings. She is senior priestess and co-founder of Mother Grove Goddess Temple and the Coalition of Earth Religions/CERES, both in Asheville, NC.

Her essays are featured in several anthologies and she writes a regular column for Witches and Pagans Magazine. Her book *Staubs and Ditchwater* debuted in 2012 and the companion volume *Asfidity and Mad-Stones* was published in Oct. 2015. *Embracing Willendorf: A Witch's Way of Loving Your Body to Health and Fitness* launched in May, 2017. *Earth Works: Ceremonies in Tower Time* debuted in June 2018. Byron is currently at work on *Gnarled Talisman: Old Wild Magics of the Motherland* and *The Ragged Wound: Tending the Soul of Appalachia.*

Caroline Selles is a veterinarian, reiki practitioner, poet and painter. A self-taught intuitive artist, Caroline began painting as a way of healing thru decades of physical and emotional trauma and illness. What began as a meditative practice with a desire to see more diversity of form and culture in art, has become a spiritual and healing practice and the pathway to finding Goddess and reclaiming her own suppressed cultural inheritance and feminine power. Essential themes of her art and poems include reclaiming female empowerment, female divinity and diversity, integration after trauma and nature as Goddess imagery. Born in Valencia, Spain, she currently resides in the United States. She can be found on social media as @thegoddesswithinart or at https://thegoddesswithinart.square.site/.

Catherine Hale is an embodied trauma coach, educator and guide specialising in sex, love, and business who believes in the power of post-traumatic growth. A heartfelt entrepreneur, Catherine is the creator of the Thrive in Life Coaching Program, which has supported 100's of courageous people to shift from surviving to Thriving in their lives. Her Thrive in Business Coaching Program is for heart centred coaches and entrepreneurs wanting to Thrive in Business and to dedicate their lives to create positive and sustainable change in the world. Her successful Trauma Awareness Training has been taken by participants in over 15 countries worldwide and continues to bridge the gap in the therapeutic community – offering trauma-informed practices and perspectives where previously absent. She is passionate about shifting the experience of menopause into one that's culturally held knowing that we need to address this shift from both a personal and systemic perspective. As a qualified trauma coach, sexological bodyworker, Trauma Release Exercises practitioner, and post-menopausal woman she writes a about a range of topics through the trauma informed lens: sex, love, relationships, menopause, women's pelvic health, and post traumatic growth.

With a lifelong passion for the natural world she lives in Devon, UK by the river Dart with her cat Simba and can be found deepening her connection to nature while exploring ancient pathways in Dartmoor National Park.

Claire Dorey. Goldsmiths: BA Hons Fine Art.

Main Employment: Journalist and Creative, UK and overseas. Artist: Most notable group show; Pillow Talk at the Tate Modern. Included in the Pillow Talk Book.

Curator: 3 x grass roots SLWA exhibitions and educational events on the subject of Female Empowerment, showcasing female artists, academic speeches and local musicians. Silence Is Over – Raising awareness on violence towards women; Ex Voto – Existential Mexican Art Therapy; Heo – Female empowerment in the self-portrait.

Extra study: Suppressed Female History: History of the Goddess; Accessing Creative Wisdom; Sound and Breath Work; Reiki Master; Colour Therapy; Hand Mudras; Reflexology; Sculpture. Teaching Workshops: Sculpture and Drawing.

Dale Allen is a veteran of corporate, creative and commercial communications. Her extensive resume includes hundreds of voice-over, on-camera, theater and live presentation projects. Dale was honored to twice present to the United Nations Commission on the Status of Women, her one-woman show, In Our Right Minds™, Guiding Women to Their Strength as Leaders, Leading Men to Strength Without Armor. Her encore was requested by the Vice President of the Commission, Ambassador Carlos Enrique Garcia Gonzales. In October 2021, she presented her new film version of the piece to the Parliament of the World's Religions. She has brought her talents to scores of audiences – across the U.S., into Canada, and from Kauai to Dubai. Described as having the energy of "a Cape Canaveral lift-off," she thoroughly engages and inspires her audience, which ranges from highly educated corporate leaders to teenage girls seeking their place in the world.

Deborah A. Meyerriecks is a retired NYC Medic, solitary witch, and community priestess who has been honored to share her story with you. Her early crone years finds her teaching, writing, learning, and exploring the Northwest of Arizona. A strong advocate for productive shadow work, she has been called to facilitate others to find their own path by holding space for them to journey and holding a lantern in the dark to help them find their way back to themselves. A returning contributor to Girl God Anthologies you can read her work in *Warrior Queen: Answering the Call of The Morrigan, Just As I Am: Hymns Affirming The Divine Female*, and *Re-Membering with Goddess*. Her own book, *Macha and the Medic: Service and Priesthood on the Frontlines of Life*, is a work in progress. She can be reached though her website: www.WillowMoonConsulting.com and by email at WillowMoon@yahoo.com

Dee Mulrooney (Growler) is an Irish artist living and working in Berlin. Raised in a working-class suburb on the Northside of Dublin in a country dominated by Catholicism and the patriarchy there was little room for artistic freedom.

Dee challenges these old paradigms with her alter-ego "Growler", an 80-year-old drum banging, shamanic giant Vulva from the inner city of Dublin. Growler facilitates healing and transmutation through storytelling, song and filthy jokes. She is a shadow worker who fits straight to the heart of taboo and takes us on a journey that only one generation ago would have seen her locked up. http://deirdre-mulrooney.com/

Dr. Denise Renye is a licensed clinical psychologist, certified sexologist, consultant and holistic coach, certified yoga therapist, and psychedelic integrationist. She has specialized training in and has worked directly with people in the areas of sexuality, relationships, embodiment, states of consciousness, psychedelic integration and intimacy. She holds a master's degree in Human Sexuality from Widener University (Philadelphia), as well as a master's degree and a Doctoral degree in Clinical Psychology from the California Institute of Integral Studies (San Francisco).

Dr. Denise is certified as a sexologist through the American College of Sexologists. She was in the first cohort to graduate from the Center for Psychedelic Therapies and Research (CPTR) at CIIS and provides psychedelic integration individually and in group settings, utilizing trauma-informed and somatics approaches. She has studied embodied spiritual practices nationally and internationally through research and experiential learning and has conducted and published research on embodied psycho-spirituality.

Elizabeth Woolfenden is a Mother, an Artist and a 'Midlife Midwife' living in The Alpujarras, Spain. Born in London in 1971, she is a mother of two, not yet teenaged, trilingual children. Her background includes midwifery, women's work, art and performance, teaching, music, and meditation.

Amongst other things, she has worked as a clown in hospitals, an independent midwife, a music teacher at the only Buddhist primary school in the UK, a jet set supernanny for billionaires, and a photographer.

She is now a Midlife Midwife! She coaches women who are ready to engage deeply and creatively with the menopause as a rite of passage. When it comes to her own life path, Lizzie has made radical choices; home-birthing, free-birthing, home-schooling, unschooling, living in different countries, living in nature, off-grid. She has often made life-changing decisions (often at lightning speed) by listening to her intuition and knowing when it's time to hold on, when it's time to jump. You can find her Midlife Soul Sisters group on Facebook or on Instragram @midlife.soul.sisters.

Ger Moane is a writer, psychologist, and shamanic practitioner who lives in Ireland and loves to visit sacred sites and sit in circle to honour the energy of Goddesses and the Celtic wheel of the year. She is fascinated by ancient Goddess spirituality, and by Newgrange, which was built 5,000 years ago and is named after the Goddess Boann. Her forthcoming novel *(Winter Sun)* is set at that time and imagines a pre-patriarchal world where humans live in harmony with Earth and sky. Her writing has been published in anthologies such as *Soul Seers, an Irish Anthology of Celtic Shamanism*, and *Goddesses of Ireland, Ancient Wisdom for Modern Women*, as well as in magazines such as Network Magazine and Eisteach.

Hayley Arrington is a poet and mythologist. Her writings have appeared in various publications, most recently in SageWoman magazine (issue 96), *In Defiance of Oppression: The Legacy of Boudicca* and *Circe's Cauldron: Pagan Poems and Tales of Magic and Witchcraft*. She believes that myth is a verdant landscape where we can feel the Goddesses of old in the present. Current projects include writing an Arthurian fantasy novel, completing a devotional poetry book for Hera, and creating an oracle deck. Hayley is from the greater Los Angeles area, where she lives her sun-drenched days with her husband and son. Find out more and read her Arthurian Witch blog at loathlylady.wordpress.com.

Janet Guastavino was born in San Francisco, California—one of the most delightful happenstances of her life. Growing up, she spent most summers with her grandmothers, above and below the great divide between Russian Hill and North Beach.

While other children played sports and Barbie, Janet enjoyed splashing in the shores of Aquatic Park (after which the North Beach grandmother would rub her raw, trying to remove every grain of sand, so none of it would cross her doorstep.) Three blocks above, she would go to help the other grandmother tend her bountiful garden, taking breaks from weeding by resting in the gentle shade of her fig tree.

When Janet was young, she wrote songs. As a crone, she writes poems. Whether music or verse, she enjoys the process of writing, particularly when it captures the essence of the souls she has known—her grandmothers among the best of them.

Jude Lally. Artist and Cultural Activist, Jude is rooted in the inspiration of her Ancestral Mothers honoring this relationship through art, ritual and storytelling. She uses old traditions to meet modern needs, such a keening, which along with ritual allows a cathartic expression of honoring grief.

She teaches courses from her annual Cailleach Circle exploring her folklore, to the tradition and practice of Keening to Creating a Meaningful Menopause. She also offers pilgrimages to the Isle of

Eigg. She gained her MSc Masters Degree in Human Ecology at the University of Strathclyde (Glasgow, Scotland) in partnership with the Center for Human Ecology.

Visit her website at www.pathoftheancestralmothers.com

On the cusp of cronehood, **Judith Murphy** is an artist ready to embrace the next phase of life with enthusiasm and humor. In her art, she portrays the crone as powerful and confident and rejects the Western world's idea that aging is diminishing. She has seen that the patriarchy wants us to value youth and ignore our elders' wisdom and knowledge but feels that growing older is a privilege we should cherish and savor. Her most recent work, Quarantine Collages, was a collaboration between neighbors and friends started during the fears and unknowns of Covid 19, a creative way to connect during the pandemic isolation. Judith lives in Philadelphia, Pennsylvania, with her husband and three feline companions.

Kaia Tingley is a writer, artist, podcaster, digital strategy nerd, and sometimes hot-tempered supernova with a wild, free soul. You can find her on Instagram or on LinkedIn. https://www.instagram.com/muse.of.creativity https://www.linkedin.com/in/kaiamaeve

Karen Storminger has been a practicing polytheist pagan most of her life. Her interests and practices include a mix of paganism, healing practices and personal study and practice with The Morrigan. She is an active member of the Connecticut Wiccan and Pagan Network and The Tuatha De Morrigan groups. A teacher and a healer in all aspects of her life, Karen believes that living itself is an act of devotion and walks through each day with the Goddess at her back, by her side and always in her heart. Karen has been writing poetry of all kinds since an early age and blogs periodically: https://thecrowandthedragonfly.wordpress.com

Kat Shaw prides herself on breaking through the stereotypical views of beauty that have been cast upon society by the media, having made her name painting the glorious reality that is a woman's body. Her nude studies of real women garnered unprecedented popularity within only a few short months, as women were crying out for themselves to be portrayed in art, rather than the airbrushed images of the perfection of the female form that are so rife in today's culture.

After graduating with a fine art degree, Kat achieved a successful full-time teaching career for 14 years, and continues to teach art part-time whilst passionately pursuing her mission of world domination by empowering as many women as possible to reach their fullest potential by embracing their bodies and loving themselves wholeheartedly.

Kat spreads her inspirational magic through her artwork, her Wellbeing business "Fabulously Imperfect" and her dedication to Goddess energy. Reiki is a huge part of her life, and as a Reiki Master, Kat is committed to sharing Reiki, teaching Usui, Angelic and Karuna Reiki, and channelling Reiki energy through her artwork to uplift and heal.

As a Sister of Avalon, Kat also works directly with her Goddess consciousness, connecting to Goddess and Priestess energy and translating it into Divine Feminine infused paintings to inspire women and spread Goddess love.

Kat is also mum to a gorgeous teenage daughter… and is a belly dancer and an avid pioneer to improve the lives of rescue animals.

Katrina Stadler is an artist who lives in Christchurch and is currently studying Bachelor of Design (Applied Visual Arts) at Ara Institute of Canterbury. She is inspired by the work of many women artists, particularly when they are making a statement about the experience of living in a woman's body or aspects of a woman's inner or outer life. Katrina is a Art of Allowing facilitator, and has facilitated women's painting and creativity workshops.

Her paintings start out as play on the canvas and then intuitively seeing and feeling what is calling to come forth, and mostly that has been feminine forms.

2020 – 2021 Bachelor of Design (Applied Visual Arts) 2020 – Year 1 Contextual Studies prize

2020 – Solo exhibition The Creatrix. Methven Memorial Hall. Canterbury

2018 – Joint exhibition Muses and Madonnas, The Feminine as Creatrix. Pumanawa Gallery Christchurch Arts Centre.

2017-2019 – Painting and creativity workshop facilitator 2017 – Certified Art of Allowing facilitator

Her website is The Art of Feminine Embodiment with Katrina Leah www.katrinaleah.com.

Kay Louise Aldred (www.kaylouisealdred.com) is a researcher, writer and teacher, who catalyses individual, institutional and collective evolution – through education, embodiment and creativity – amalgamating metacognition, intuition and instinct.

Her own books include *Mentorship with Goddess: Growing Sacred Womanhood, Making Love with the Divine: Sacred, Ecstatic, Erotic, Experiences* and *Somatic Shamanism: Your Fleshy Knowing as the Tree of Life*.

Kay and her husband Dan Aldred also have co-authored a book together: *Embodied Education: Creating Safe Space for Learning, Facilitating and Sharing*.

Laura Valenti is a Moon dancer, nomad at heart, lover of community, music, drums, wilderness and ceremony, Laura was born in Italy, where she learnt about good food, hospitality and colourful swearing. She is a qualified Movement Medicine dance teacher and facilitator.

In her early thirties, she was diagnosed with Non-Hodgkins Lymphoma. While undergoing treatments for cancer she committed to deepening her exploration of movement as medicine. Her curiosity and passion for learning led her over two decades to study formally and informally many modalities, including the Andean cosmology, Theta healing, Polarity therapy, animism, laughter yoga and Earth-based spirituality. She is a qualified sound & voice therapist, somatic & trauma-sensitive coach and trained professionally in physical theatre and clowning.

Laura's background is in law, sociology of migration and human rights. She shared her work internationally with indigenous communities, people in drug and alcohol rehabilitation, refugees, women victim of domestic violence and vulnerable children.

Lauren Raine, MFA, has been creating visual and performance art about the Great Mother since the early 80's. She studied sacred mask traditions in Bali, and exhibited at Buka Creati Gallery in Ubud, Bali. Her collection of "contemporary temple masks" devoted to worldwide stories of the sacred feminine, The Masks of the Goddess, traveled throughout the U.S. for over 20 years used by dancers, ritualists, and storytellers. Venues included the Chapel of Sacred Mirrors, the International Mask Symposium, the New College of California, and the Parliament of World Religions. In 2007 she received a Fellowship with the Alden Dow Creativity Center at Northwood University and a Puffin Grant for her "Spider Woman" Community Arts Project. In 2009 she was resident artist at the Henry Luce Center for the Arts at Wesley Theological Seminary in Washington, DC. Currently she works in ceramic sculpture and teaches at the Tucson Clay Co-op. www.laurenraine.com / www.masksofthegoddess.com

Leonor Murciano-Luna, Ph.D., integrative doctor, healer, spiritual teacher, mystic, sacred sound artist and author of Birth of the Conscious Feminine, Evolution of our Feminine Soul, founder of Feminine Path APP, School of Conscious Feminine Medicine & Conscious Feminine Revolution PODCAST. Dedicated to embodying our Soul 's expression fully as we heal Feminine trauma, personally, and collectively.

Liliana Kleiner Ph.D. is a visual artist born in Argentina and raised in Israel. She divides her time living and working in Jerusalem and in North and South America.Liliana is known for her visionary oil paintings and her Earthy woodcuts which convey her vision of the "Spirit of the Earth." Her work is Visual Poetry from a Feminine Spiritual perspective.

Liliana creates her own organic hand-made paper, and had published two art books—*The Song of Lilith* (2007) and *The Song of Songs, Jerusalem* (2010). She has produced art films—*Lilith and the Tree* (1993) and *Lesbian Tango* (2006) and works with performance arts and dance.

In addition to her career as an artist, Liliana has a Ph.D. in clinical Psychology, and specializes in Jungian Dream Analysis. Her work is in galleries and private collections in America and Israel, and can be seen in her site: www.lilianakleiner.com

Dr Lynne Sedgmore CBE is a Priestess of Avalon, Poetess, retired Chief Executive, soul coach and Priestess healer. She is founder and tutor of the Goddess Luminary Leadership Wheel trainings, a unique combination of liberating leadership, feminism and Goddess spirituality offered through the Glastonbury Goddess Temple. Her new book *The Goddess Luminary Leadership Wheel* will be published by John Hunt, Changemakers Imprint, in 2022.

Lynne has spent her professional career teaching and leading in the UK Further Education sector. Her roles included CEO of 157 Group, Chief Executive of the national Centre for Excellence in Leadership, and Principal of Guildford College.

Her three poetry collections are *Enlivenment* (Chrysalis Press 2013), *Healing through the Goddess* (TheaSpeaks Press 2017) and *Crone* (TheaSpeaks Press 2019). She has published a range of articles on spirituality and leadership.

Lynne has 3 daughters and 2 granddaughters and lives in Glastonbury UK.

Mary Lane is an elder whose path has been devoted to transformation. Throughout her journey she has transformed her relationship with the patriarchal version of sexuality, food, the feminine, Mother Earth, and now death. For the last 30 years she has supported others, as she has navigated her own archetypal journey. She has learned the importance of reclaiming death as a sacred passage, that is woven into the fabric of the natural world, we are very much a part of, and affects every aspect of life.

Deepening her role as a crone, she has taken her seat in alignment with the wisdom she has garnered, and is devoting her time as a death doula, and her program, Making Friends With Death. Mary is dedicated to supporting herself and others to transform our relationship with death. www.divinenourishment.net

Mary Saracino is a novelist, memoir writer, and poet. Her most recent novel, *Heretics: A Love Story* (2014) was published by Pearlsong Press. Her novel, *The Singing of Swans* (Pearlsong Press 2006) was named a 2007 Lambda Literary Awards finalist in the Spirituality category. For more information about Mary and her work, visit www.marysaracino.com and http://www.pearlsong.com/mary_saracino.htm

Molly Remer, MSW, **D.Min**, is a priestess facilitating women's circles, seasonal rituals, and family ceremonies in central Missouri. Molly and her husband Mark co-create Story Goddesses at Brigid's Grove. Molly is the author of nine books, including *Walking with Persephone, Whole and Holy, Womanrunes,* and the *Goddess Devotional*. She is the creator of the devotional experience #30DaysofGoddess and she loves savoring small magic and everyday enchantment.

Nikki Wardwell Sleath, MA, a direct descendant of one of the colonial citizens of Salem accused and killed for Witchcraft, is a lifelong witch herself. Originally a physical therapist by trade, her foray into integrative health and healing and her spiritual practice and formal training as a witch have led her to a long-term, full-time career teaching magick and leading ritual in her order, the

Society of Witchcraft and Old Magick. She is a healer, hypnotherapist, dream work facilitator, author, wife and mom to two wonderful young adults.

Nuit Moore is a ceremonial creatrix, ritual artist, witch and eco-feminist activist whose work has served the return of the Goddess to the collective consciousness. As a priestess, she has been teaching and offering women's ceremonies for almost 30 years, and is also ordained as a Priestess within the Fellowship of Isis.

Nuit has been a visionary voice and red thread weaver of the Blood Mysteries and an activist of the eco-menstruation movement since 1991. Much of her path is rooted in women's rites/rights, which is also embodied in her work as an herbalist of the Wise Woman tradition. Having now reached her 50's, Nuit embraces the alchemy at hand, the curving path of her journey, and is excited to see where it leads her. She is currently directing her focus more deeply to her work as a creatrix and ritual artist of multiple forms, to her ancestral lineages, as well as towards an evolving and expanded service to Dea Madre.

She can be found via Instagram @nuitmoore and she has a new website in progress, information of which will be accessible via her IG bio when complete. Her currently available ceremonial sculptures as well as her herbal offerings are available via Etsy at www.shaktistudios.etsy.com

Pat Daly (editor) is a mother of three daughters, and proud grandma. A published author/writer on career and job search issues, Pat lives in Portland, Oregon. She has edited all of the Girl God Books from the beginning.

Rhonda Melanson has been published in several print and online magazines, including: The Wild Word, Juniper, The Boxcar Poetry Review, Quill's, Philadelphia Poets, Ascent Aspirations, Lummox, and the Windsor Review. In 2011, she published a chapbook called *Gracenotes* with Beret Days Press. She was most recently published in *She Summons: Why Goddess Feminism, Activism and Spirituality* by Mago Books.

Rebekah Myers is dedicated to opening doors of understanding on behalf of women everywhere. She is the founder/facilitator of Sacred Sisters Full Moon Circle, which serves as a virtual Facebook and Instagram public page, a private Facebook group for women, and an actual women's circle that meets in-person. For International Women's Day in March of 2018, Rebekah was honored to have been one of five women recognized by KSL as Utah's most inspirational women.

Through her social anthropologist parents, Rebekah spent memorable time with the Iroquois (a matrilineal people) of Six Nations Reserve in Ontario, Canada. This experience significantly informed her life for the good. Rebekah has had a life-long interest in and passion for folklore, mythology, and ancient history, and has spent significant time in these worlds. Although Rebekah formally came later in life to women's spirituality, she has found such fulfillment on this path, that there is no turning back. As a writer, teacher, director, award-winning singer/performer/actress, mother, grandmother, and wedding officiator, Rebekah works to empower, enlighten, and uplift women and their brothers. She knows it is possible to heal the wounds of patriarchy and live with depth, meaning, and joy.

Sarah Miller is a Teacher of the Four Seasons Journey and MoonSong (Menstrual Wellness) Workshop for the School of Shamanic Womancraft. She works with women in recreating mytho-poetic and embodied stories of their rites of passage and teaches the fundamentals of menstrual wellness. Through her business Embodiments Dance Sarah offers seasonal dance celebrations, drum making workshops and women's circles. Sarah is an emerging playwright, and filmmaker. Her latest short film, Giving Voice to Menopause made with co-directors Libby Chow and Vanessa Chapple recently screened at Female Voices Rock Film Festival New York.

Sharon Smith is a writer, ghost writer, editor, and proofreader with a passion for helping women reconnect with their Authentic Selves and Voices. She loves & honors the Great Mother in all Her many forms, and has a deep connection to Nature. She identifies as a Green Witch and follows an eclectic spiritual path that is a blending of Native American and Celtic Teachings, both in her ancestral line.

Stella Webb is a mother, stepmother, grandmother, wife, business owner, writer, pagan priestess, meditation facilitator, Reiki Master Teacher, nature lover... and crone.

Dr. Stephanie Mines is the author of five books that reflect over three decades of research as a neuroscientist. She has investigated shock and trauma as a survivor, a professional, a clinical researcher, and healthcare provider. Her nonprofit The TARA Approach is instrumental in the systemic change she promotes as a Regenerative Health paradigm.

Dr. Mines also developed Climate Change & Consciousness to facilitate inner transformation for grounded climate action. Climate Change & Consciousness serves an international and intergenerational community of visionary activists.

In addition, Dr. Mines is an award-winning poet. Her poetry has been published in anthologies and in chapbooks. Dr. Mines' latest book, *Memoir of An Embryologist: How I Discovered the Secret of Resilience*, will be released in 2023 from Inner Traditions/Sacred Planet Books.

Sue Lobo is the author of five books of her own & co-author with worldwide poets in another twenty-one publications. She has also participated in poetry competitions in Gibraltar & Spain. She is married to a Spaniard, with two grown up sons & two grandsons & presently lives in Spain. Her book of poetry about death & dying called "The Last Dance" was reviewed on Italian television & has been used to comfort the bereaved in hospices & also used at funerals. She champions women & their fight for equality around the world & especially the age of women's Cronedom. As a child she grew up in the Kalahari Desert in Botswana among the Bushmen who taught her the beauty & magic of nature & unity of the tribe. She was born in England & has lived in many countries which has influenced her work. Sue writes poetry daily & can be followed on Facebook.

Suzanne Taylor-Torres is a traditional Usui Reiki Master. She began her studies on Long Island, NY in 1995. She holds certifications in Light Work with White Light Seminars, Hypnosis and Past Life Regression, and has studied Medicine Wheel and Full Moon Ceremony. A move to Tucson, AZ brought training in: LED Light Treatment, Essential Oils and supplements, and aromatic touch for wellness.

While living in Sedona, she added the titles of Minister to her services, and Author, of two books: "Journey to Now", a spiritual biography, and "Basic Steps to Law of Attraction", outlining manifesting principles.

Suzanne worked with UFOlogist David Sereda/Light Stream Technology pendants, and trained with Elizabeth Wilcock Priestess Path Lineages of Light. In 2021, she brought certification to the Hawaiian practice of Ho'oponopono. Suzanne was an elementary and special education teacher for over 30 years with a BA in Elementary Ed. and MS in Special Ed.

Trista Hendren founded Girl God Books in 2011 to support a necessary unraveling of the patriarchal worldview of divinity. Her first book—*The Girl God*, a children's picture book—was a response to her own daughter's inability to see herself reflected in the divine. Since then, she has published more than 50 books with hundreds of contributors from across the globe. Originally from Portland, Oregon, she now lives in Bergen, Norway. You can learn more about her projects at www.thegirlgod.com

Trista's Acknowledgments

First, I would like to acknowledge my co-editors. My mother, **Pat Daly**, has edited each and every one of my books. There would be no Girl God Books without her enormous contributions. I was also thrilled to work with **Kay Louise Aldred** again on this project, who came up with the brilliant idea for this book.

A thousand thanks to **H. Byron Ballard** for writing such a phenomenal foreword and essay. You outdid yourself—and that's saying a lot.

Love and appreciation for my beloved Sister **Sharon Smith** for carefully editing my pieces. You have no idea how much this helped me.

Tremendous gratitude to **Kat Shaw** for allowing us to feature her gorgeous painting as the cover art.

Many thanks to all the contributors, whose art and writings made this anthology so special.

Enormous appreciation to my husband **Anders Løberg,** who created the book cover and helped with website updates. Your love, support and many contributions make my life beautiful.

Lastly, I would like to thank my dear sisters Tamara Albanna, Susan Morgaine, Jessica Bahr, Jeanette Bjørnsen, Kay Louise Aldred, Sharon Smith, Arlene Bailey, Arna Baartz, Kat Shaw, Tammy Nedrebø-Skurtveit, Lisa Belfiore, and Alyscia Cunningham for always being right there to cheer me on in the spirit of true sisterhood.

Thank you to all our readers and Girl God supporters over the years. We love and appreciate you!

Kay's Acknowledgments

I'd like to thank the truth-tellers, the women who are courageously and authentically sharing their menopause journeys, offering their wisdom, inspiration and support to others as they do.

I'm grateful to and for the wisdom of my ancestors, the Grandmothers of my lineage.

Gratitude to Dark Goddess and the intelligence of embodiment, of our womb and the beauty of aged skin and wrinkles.

Thank you to for birthing Girl God and her tireless trial blazing commitment to **Trista Hendren** woman and the sacred feminine. Thank you for believing in me and your yes.

Huge appreciation to my co-editor **Pat Daly** and to **Kat Shaw** for the bold and inspiring cover art.

And finally huge love and appreciation for my husband **Dan** and his love, his endless curiosity, encouragement and avid engagement with my creativity and passions.

Upcoming Girl God Books

Wounded Feminine: Grieving with Goddess – Edited by Claire Dorey, Trista Hendren, and Pat Daly

Asherah: Roots of the Mother Tree – Edited by Claire Dorey, Janet Rudolph, Pat Daly and Trista Hendren

Sacred Breasts – Edited by Barbara O'Meara and Trista Hendren

The Wisdom of Cerridwen: Transforming in Her Cosmic Brew – Edited by Emma Clark, Trista Hendren, and Pat Daly

Lady of the Forge: Stories and Art Dedicated to the Goddess Brigid – Edited by Isca Johnson, Trista Hendren, and Pat Daly

Songs of Solstice: Goddess Carols – Edited by Trista Hendren, Sharon Smith and Pat Daly

Rainbow Goddess – Celebrating Neurodiversity – Edited by Kay Louise Aldred, Tamara Albanna, Trista Hendren and Pat Daly

Women's Sovereignty and Body Autonomy Beyond Roe v. Wade – Edited by Arlene Bailey, Pat Daly, Sharon Smith and Trista Hendren

Kali Rising: Sacred Rage – Edited by C. Ara Campbell, Jaclyn Cherie, Pat Daly, and Trista Hendren

Pain Perspectives: Finding Meaning in the Fire – Edited by Kay Louise Aldred, Trista Hendren and Pat Daly

Making Love with the Divine: Sacred, Ecstatic, and Erotic Experiences – Kay Louise Aldred

For recent writings and news of upcoming publications, join us on Patreon @girlgodbooks!

If you enjoyed this book, please consider writing a brief review on StoryGraph, Amazon and/or Goodreads.

We LOVE photos of our readers with Girl God Books! Tag @girlgodbooks on social media – or email them to support@girlgod.org.